PLANT BASED DIET COOKBOOK FOR SENIORS

A comprehensive Guide to Healthy Eating

By

Hector Wiggins

Table of Contents

INTRODUCTION

In the quiet neighborhood of Green Haven, nestled among the rustling leaves and blossoming gardens, lived Mrs. Eleanor Thompson, a spirited senior with a contagious zest for life. As the aroma of freshly baked apple pie wafted from her kitchen, a secret to her vibrant well-being lingered in the air—a plant-based diet.

The genesis of this cookbook is rooted in Mrs. Thompson's journey. Turning the pages of her life, you'll discover the transformative power of plant-based eating, especially tailored for the golden years. In her cozy kitchen, where laughter echoed alongside the clinking of utensils, she effortlessly created dishes that not only tantalized the taste buds but also nourished her body with the vitality needed to embrace each day.

Allow me to extend an invitation to you, dear reader, to embark on this culinary adventure designed specifically for seniors. Picture yourself wandering through a farmer's market, selecting vibrant produce that will soon find its way into delectable recipes crafted with love and wisdom.

In the chapters that follow, we'll explore the essence of plant-based nutrition for seniors—a harmonious symphony of flavors and nutrients that beckons you to savor each bite. From energizing breakfasts to comforting soups, hearty dinners, and guilt-free desserts, every recipe is a homage to the richness of life that age should never diminish.

This cookbook is not just a collection of recipes; it's a companion on your journey toward enhanced well-being. Alongside nutritional insights and practical tips, you'll find stories of seniors who have embraced plant-based living, defying stereotypes and celebrating the joy that comes with embracing a healthier lifestyle.

So, let's step into Mrs. Thompson's kitchen together, where the warmth of compassion meets the vibrancy of plant-powered living. Let this cookbook be your guide to unlocking the potential for a healthier, more joyful chapter in your life. Welcome to the "Plant-Based Diet Cookbook for Seniors," where the journey is as delightful as the destination.

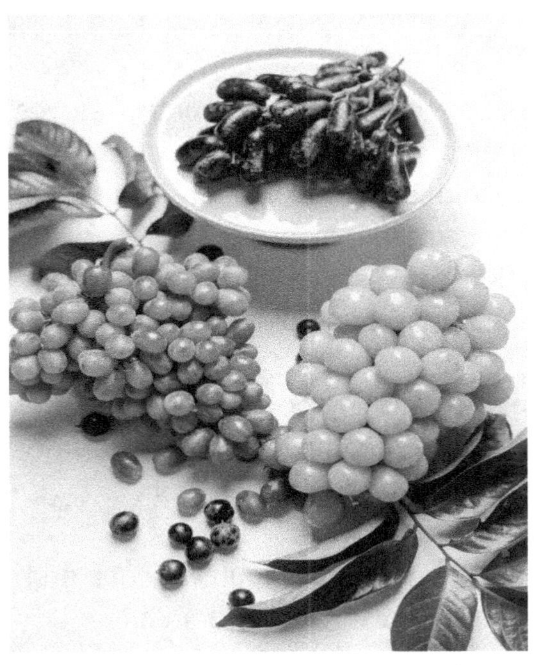

1 Welcome to a Plant-Powered Journey

Welcome to a Plant-Powered Journey" serves as an invitation to embark on a transformative exploration into the world of plant-based living. This phrase is more than a mere greeting; it encapsulates the essence of adopting a lifestyle centered around plant-based nutrition.

In the context of a plant-powered journey, the term "plant-powered" implies drawing sustenance and vitality primarily from plant-derived sources, such as fruits, vegetables, whole grains, legumes, nuts, and seeds. It signifies a shift away from an animal-centric diet toward one that prioritizes the diverse and nutrient-rich offerings of the plant kingdom.

The notion of a "journey" conveys the idea that adopting a plant-based lifestyle is not just a destination but an ongoing process of discovery, learning, and growth. It suggests that individuals are embarking on a path with the potential for personal transformation, improved well-being, and a positive impact on the environment.

"Welcome to a Plant-Powered Journey" sets the tone for exploration, curiosity, and a willingness to embrace new perspectives on food, health, and sustainability. It extends an inclusive invitation, encouraging individuals to step into this lifestyle with an open heart and a sense of excitement for the possibilities that lie ahead.

This welcoming phrase is often found at the beginning of resources, such as cookbooks, guides, or websites dedicated to plant-based living. It serves as an introduction to the philosophy, principles, and benefits of choosing plant-based foods, inviting individuals to join a community that values health, compassion, and a connection to the natural world.

2 Why Plant-Based Eating for Seniors

Why Plant-Based Eating for Seniors" delves into the compelling reasons behind choosing a plant-based diet tailored specifically for individuals in their golden years. This exploration goes beyond a mere dietary preference, touching on the unique health considerations and benefits that make plant-based eating an excellent choice for seniors.

Nutrient Density and Absorption:
Plant-based foods are rich in vitamins, minerals, and antioxidants, offering seniors a nutrient-dense approach to support overall health. Improved nutrient absorption becomes crucial as aging bodies may experience challenges in assimilating nutrients effectively.

Heart Health and Cholesterol Management:
A plant-based diet has been associated with cardiovascular health benefits. Seniors can benefit from lower saturated fats found in plant foods, aiding in cholesterol management and reducing the risk of heart-related issues.

Weight Management and Metabolic Health:
Seniors often face challenges related to weight management and metabolic changes. Plant-based eating promotes a balanced approach to calories, fiber-rich foods, and plant compounds that support metabolism and weight maintenance.

Digestive Health and Fiber Intake:
Fiber-rich plant foods contribute to digestive health, alleviating concerns such as constipation. A plant-based diet naturally provides the fiber needed for digestive regularity, promoting gut health and overall well-being.

Bone Health and Nutrient Synergy:
While dairy is often associated with bone
health, plant-based sources like leafy greens,
fortified plant milks, and nuts contribute
essential nutrients such as calcium and vitamin
D. These nutrients work synergistically to
support bone strength.

Inflammation Reduction:
Chronic inflammation is linked to various
age-related diseases. Plant-based foods
possess anti-inflammatory properties,
potentially aiding in reducing inflammation and
mitigating the risk of inflammatory-related
conditions.

Cognitive Health and Antioxidants:
Antioxidant-rich fruits and vegetables play a
role in cognitive health. Seniors may find
benefits in consuming a variety of colorful plant
foods that support brain function and may
contribute to a lower risk of cognitive decline.

Hydration and Nutrient-Rich Fluids:
Many plant-based foods, such as fruits and vegetables, have high water content, aiding in hydration. For seniors, maintaining proper hydration is crucial, and plant-based foods can contribute to overall fluid intake.

Sustainability and Environmental Impact:
Plant-based eating aligns with sustainability efforts, promoting a diet that has a lower environmental impact. This consideration extends beyond personal health to contributing to a healthier planet for future generations.

Adaptable and Flexible:
Plant-based eating is adaptable to various dietary preferences and restrictions. Seniors can tailor their plant-based approach to suit individual tastes, cultural considerations, and specific health needs.

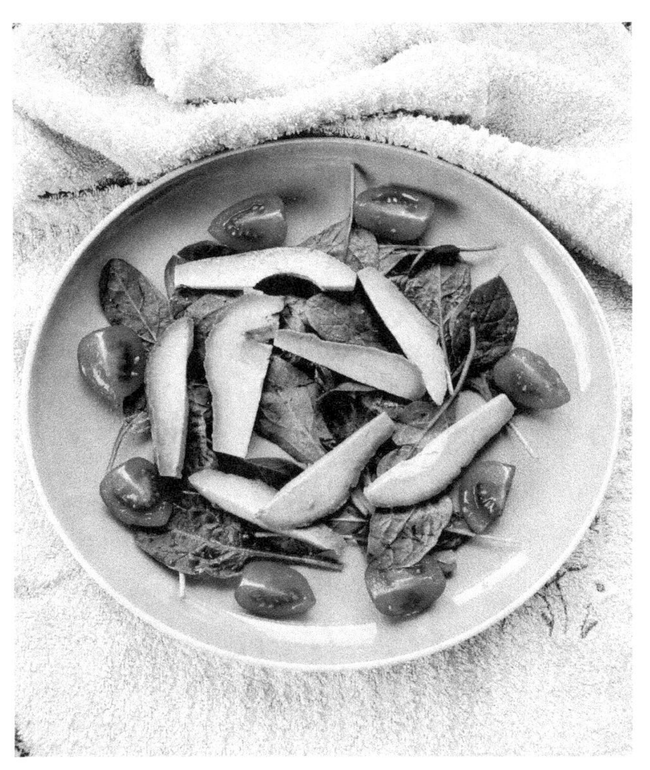

3 Tips for Success on a Plant-Based Diet

Embracing a plant-based diet can be a rewarding journey for your health and the environment. Here are some tips for success on a plant-based diet:

Educate Yourself:
Learn about plant-based nutrition to ensure you are getting a well-rounded and balanced diet. Understand the essential nutrients found in plant foods and how to meet your dietary needs.

Begin Gradually:
It's not necessary to switch to a plant-based diet all at once. Increase the amount of plant-based meals you eat each day and then progressively cut back on animal products.

Explore New Foods:
Experiment with a variety of fruits, vegetables, grains, legumes, nuts, and seeds. Trying new foods keeps your meals exciting and helps you discover flavors you enjoy.

Plan Balanced Meals:
Ensure your meals are balanced with a mix of carbohydrates, proteins, healthy fats, vitamins, and minerals. Include a variety of colorful vegetables and whole grains for optimal nutrition.

Protein-Rich Plant Foods:
Include protein-rich plant foods such as beans, lentils, tofu, tempeh, quinoa, and edamame. Combining different protein sources ensures you get a complete amino acid profile.

Read Labels:
Be mindful of processed foods and read labels to avoid hidden animal products. Look for whole, unprocessed plant foods to maximize nutritional benefits.

Stay Hydrated:
Water is essential for overall health. Ensure you stay adequately hydrated, and consider incorporating hydrating foods like fruits and vegetables into your diet.

Meal Prep and Planning:
Plan your meals in advance and consider meal prepping to make plant-based eating more convenient. Having nutritious, ready-to-go options reduces the likelihood of resorting to less healthy choices.

Vitamin B12 Supplement:
Since vitamin B12 is primarily found in animal
products, consider taking a B12 supplement or
consuming B12-fortified foods to ensure you
meet your nutritional needs.

Connect with Others:
Join plant-based communities or find friends
and family who share similar dietary choices.
Connecting with others can provide support,
recipe ideas, and encouragement.

Incorporate Diversity:
Include a diverse range of plant foods to
ensure you receive a broad spectrum of
nutrients. Eating a variety of fruits, vegetables,
and grains contributes to overall nutritional
well-being.

Be Mindful of Nutrient Intake:
Keep track of essential nutrients, especially calcium, iron, zinc, and omega-3 fatty acids. Ensure you're meeting your requirements through plant-based sources or supplements if needed.

Enjoy the Journey:
Embrace the plant-based lifestyle with a positive mindset. Enjoy the process of discovering new foods, flavors, and the positive impact your choices make on your health and the environment.

Remember that everyone's journey to a plant-based diet is unique. It's about finding what works best for you, incorporating a variety of nutrient-rich foods, and enjoying the benefits of a plant-powered lifestyle.

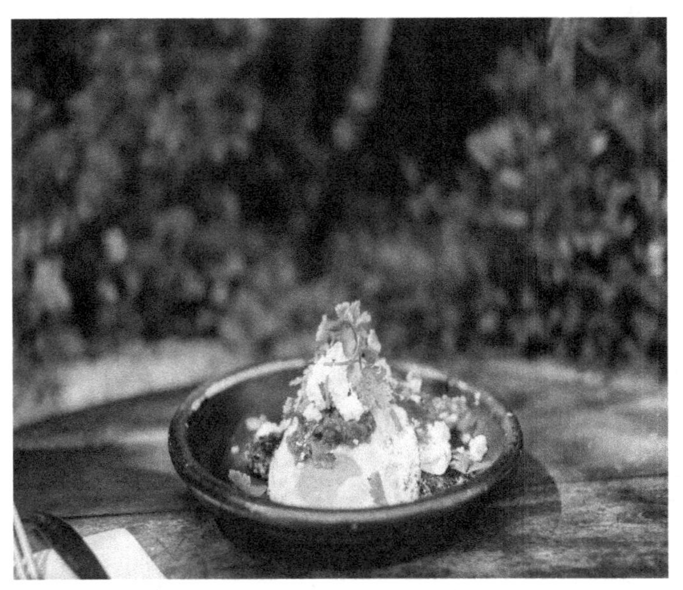

CHAPTER ONE

1 The Senior's Guide to Plant-Based Nutrition

The Senior's Guide to Plant-Based Nutrition" serves as a comprehensive resource tailored to meet the unique dietary needs and considerations of older individuals embracing a plant-based lifestyle. This section delves into key aspects of plant-based nutrition, offering valuable insights to seniors seeking to optimize their health and well-being through mindful dietary choices.

Understanding Plant-Based Nutrients:
This part of the guide illuminates the array of essential nutrients abundant in plant-based foods.

It provides a detailed exploration of vitamins, minerals, antioxidants, and other beneficial compounds found in fruits, vegetables, grains, legumes, nuts, and seeds. Understanding these nutrients is pivotal for seniors aiming to craft a well-rounded and nourishing plant-based diet.

Addressing Common Nutritional Concerns for Seniors:
Seniors may face specific nutritional challenges, such as maintaining bone health, managing digestive issues, or ensuring adequate protein intake. The guide addresses these concerns, offering practical tips and plant-based solutions to support seniors in achieving optimal nutrition tailored to their life stage.

Building a Balanced Plant-Based Plate:
Creating a balanced plate is essential for seniors adopting a plant-based diet.

This section provides guidance on portion sizes, macronutrient distribution, and the inclusion of a variety of plant foods to ensure seniors meet their nutritional requirements. It emphasizes the importance of diversity for a wholesome and satisfying plant-based meal.

"The Senior's Guide to Plant-Based Nutrition" aims to empower older individuals with the knowledge and tools necessary to navigate the intricacies of a plant-based lifestyle. By providing targeted information on nutrient-rich foods, addressing common nutritional concerns, and offering practical tips for balanced meals, this guide becomes a trusted companion on the journey toward vibrant and healthful senior living.

1.1 **Understand Plant-Based Nutrient**

Understanding plant-based nutrients involves gaining insight into the diverse array of essential compounds derived from plant sources that contribute to overall health and well-being. Plant-based diets focus on incorporating a rich variety of fruits, vegetables, whole grains, legumes, nuts, and seeds, each offering a unique set of nutrients that play crucial roles in supporting bodily functions. Here's a breakdown of key plant-based nutrients:

Vitamins:
Vitamin A, C, and E: Abundant in fruits and vegetables, these antioxidants contribute to immune function and protect cells from oxidative stress.
Vitamin K: Found in leafy greens, it supports blood clotting and bone health.

Minerals:

Calcium: Essential for bone health, sources include fortified plant milks, leafy greens, and almonds.

Iron: Found in legumes, tofu, and dark leafy greens, supporting oxygen transport in the blood.

Zinc: Nuts, seeds, and legumes are sources that contribute to immune function.

Antioxidants:

Flavonoids, Carotenoids, and Polyphenols: These powerful compounds found in various plant foods help neutralize free radicals, protecting cells from damage.

Fiber:

Soluble and Insoluble Fiber: Abundant in whole grains, fruits, and vegetables, fiber supports digestive health, regulates blood sugar, and helps manage weight.

Proteins:
Legumes, Tofu, and Quinoa: These plant-based sources provide essential amino acids for muscle repair and overall body function.

Healthy Fats:
Omega-3 Fatty Acids: Found in flaxseeds, chia seeds, and walnuts, these fats support heart and brain health.

Phytochemicals:
Glucosinolates, Lycopene, and Anthocyanins: Plant compounds with potential health benefits, found in cruciferous vegetables, tomatoes, and berries, respectively.

.

1.2 Addressing Common Nutritional Concerns for Seniors

Addressing common nutritional concerns for seniors on a plant-based diet involves thoughtful consideration of the unique needs that come with aging. While adopting a plant-based lifestyle offers numerous health benefits, seniors may encounter specific challenges related to nutrient absorption, bone health, and other age-related factors. Here's how these concerns are addressed:

Bone Health:
Concern: Seniors are often mindful of maintaining bone health, especially regarding calcium and vitamin D intake.
Solution: The guide provides insights into plant-based sources of calcium, such as fortified plant milks, leafy greens, and nuts. Additionally, it encourages safe sun exposure for natural vitamin D synthesis.

Protein Intake:

Concern: Seniors may worry about obtaining sufficient protein for muscle maintenance and overall health.

Solution: The guide highlights protein-rich plant sources like legumes, tofu, tempeh, and quinoa, ensuring seniors meet their protein needs without relying on animal products.

Digestive Health:

Concern: Aging can sometimes lead to digestive issues, and seniors may seek advice on maintaining gut health.

Solution: The guide emphasizes the importance of fiber-rich plant foods for digestive regularity and includes tips on incorporating probiotic-rich foods like fermented plant-based options.

Nutrient Absorption:

Concern: Aging can impact nutrient absorption, raising questions about getting enough vitamins and minerals.

Solution: The guide addresses this concern by recommending a variety of nutrient-dense plant foods, often in easily digestible forms, and suggests cooking techniques to enhance nutrient bioavailability.

Hydration:
Concern: Seniors may face challenges in staying adequately hydrated, impacting overall health.
Solution: The guide encourages the consumption of hydrating plant foods, such as fruits and vegetables with high water content, to support hydration and overall well-being.

Adapting to Changes:
Concern: As seniors undergo changes in metabolism and energy levels, they may need guidance on adjusting their plant-based diet accordingly.

Solution: The guide provides insights into adapting portion sizes, choosing nutrient-dense foods, and incorporating energy-boosting snacks to meet changing nutritional needs.

Supplementation Guidance:
Concern: Seniors may wonder about the need for supplements on a plant-based diet.
Solution: The guide offers advice on plant-based supplements, such as vitamin B12, and emphasizes the importance of consulting healthcare professionals for personalized guidance.

Cognitive Health:
Concern: Maintaining cognitive function becomes a priority for seniors.
Solution: The guide introduces antioxidant-rich plant foods that support brain health and may contribute to a lower risk of cognitive decline.

1.3 **Building a Balanced Plant-Based Plate**

Building a balanced plant-based plate involves creating meals that provide a diverse array of nutrients essential for overall health and well-being. The goal is to combine different food groups, ensuring an adequate intake of proteins, carbohydrates, healthy fats, vitamins, and minerals. Here's a breakdown of how to build a well-balanced plant-based plate:

Foundation of Whole Grains:
Start with a base of whole grains like quinoa, brown rice, or whole wheat pasta. These grains provide complex carbohydrates for sustained energy and fiber for digestive health.

Ample veggies: Arrange a vibrant selection of veggies to cover half of your plate. Incorporate a diverse range of colorful vegetables, leafy greens, and cruciferous veggies to guarantee a comprehensive intake of vitamins, minerals, and antioxidants.

Protein-Rich Foods:
Incorporate plant-based protein sources such as legumes (beans, lentils), tofu, tempeh, and edamame. These proteins contribute essential amino acids for muscle maintenance and overall bodily functions.

Healthy Fats:
Add a source of healthy fats like avocados, nuts, seeds, or olive oil. These fats support nutrient absorption and provide essential fatty acids.

Plant-Based Proteins or Substitutes:
Consider including plant-based proteins or substitutes like veggie burgers, seitan, or plant-based sausages for variety and additional protein options.

Fruits for Dessert or Side:
Include fruits for dessert or as a side to add natural sweetness, fiber, and a variety of vitamins. Fresh fruits, berries, or a fruit salad are excellent choices.

Herbs and Spices:
Enhance flavor without relying on excessive salt by using herbs and spices. Fresh herbs or a sprinkle of turmeric, cumin, or garlic can elevate the taste of your dish.

Hydration:
Accompany your meal with water, herbal teas, or infused water to stay hydrated. Limit sugary drinks and opt for beverages that complement your plant-based choices.

Meal Size and Portion Control:
Pay attention to portion sizes to avoid
overeating. A balanced plate incorporates a
variety of foods without overwhelming your
calorie intake.

Nutrient Density: Choose meals that are high
in vitamins and minerals per calorie and have a
high nutrient density. To get the most nutritional
benefits, choose meals that are whole and little
processed.

Consider Nutritional Needs:
Tailor your plate to meet specific nutritional
needs, such as incorporating calcium-rich
foods for bone health and vitamin B12 sources
for energy metabolism.

CHAPTER TWO

2 Essential Kitchen Tools and Ingredients

Essential Kitchen Tools:
Blender:

Ideal for creating smoothies, soups, and sauces, providing a convenient way to incorporate fruits and vegetables into meals.

Food Processor:
A versatile tool for chopping, slicing, and dicing vegetables, making it easier for seniors to include a variety of plant-based ingredients in their recipes.

Sharp Knives:
Ensure seniors have high-quality, sharp knives
to make cutting fruits, vegetables, and
plant-based proteins safer and more efficient.

Non-Stick Cookware:
Eases cooking and cleaning, promoting
healthier cooking with less oil while preparing
plant-based meals.

Steamer Basket:
Preserves the nutritional content of vegetables
during cooking, offering a simple way to
prepare them without losing essential vitamins.

Slow Cooker:
Perfect for preparing hearty plant-based stews,
soups, and legumes, allowing for easy,
hands-off cooking.

Easy-to-Grip Utensils:
Consider utensils with ergonomic designs for comfortable handling, enhancing the cooking experience for seniors.

Measuring Cups and Spoons:
Essential for precise ingredient measurements, especially crucial when following plant-based recipes that require specific proportions.

Essential Ingredients:

Leafy Greens:
Packed with vitamins and minerals, including kale, spinach, and collard greens, providing a foundation for nutrient-rich meals.

Legumes:
Beans, lentils, and chickpeas offer plant-based protein, fiber, and various nutrients, supporting seniors' overall health.

Whole Grains:
Quinoa, brown rice, and oats provide essential carbohydrates and fiber, contributing to sustained energy levels.

Plant-Based Proteins:
Tofu, tempeh, and seitan can be versatile protein sources, adding variety and nutrition to meals.

Nuts and Seeds:
Almonds, chia seeds, and flaxseeds supply healthy fats, protein, and omega-3 fatty acids, supporting heart health.

Colorful Vegetables:
Include a variety of vibrant vegetables for a range of vitamins, minerals, and antioxidants, enhancing both flavor and nutrition.

Avocados:
A rich source of heart-healthy fats, avocados add creaminess and nutritional value to dishes.

Herbs and Spices:
Enhance flavor without relying on excessive salt, promoting a more heart-healthy approach to seasoning.

A plant-based diet for seniors should prioritize nutrient density, ease of preparation, and enjoyable flavors to support their health and well-being.

2.1 Equipping Your Plant-Powered Kitchen

Invest in Senior-Friendly Tools:
Opt for kitchen tools designed with ergonomic grips and easy-to-use features to ensure seniors can handle them comfortably. Consider lightweight yet durable materials for utensils and cookware.

User-Friendly Blender and Food Processor:
Select a blender with simple controls for smoothies and soups, and a user-friendly food processor with easy-to-assemble parts. These appliances should simplify the preparation of plant-based meals.

Adapted Cutting Solutions:
Ensure seniors have access to adaptive cutting boards and tools designed to make chopping and slicing easier. Sharp, manageable knives with safety features can enhance the overall cooking experience.

Accessible Storage Containers:
Choose containers with easy-open lids and clear markings for seniors to store prepped ingredients and leftovers conveniently. This promotes organization and makes meal preparation more efficient.

Senior-Friendly Cookware:
Invest in non-stick cookware to make cooking and cleaning hassle-free. Lightweight pans with heat-resistant handles ensure safety and ease of use.

Simple-to-Read Measuring Tools:
Opt for measuring cups and spoons with large, clear markings to aid seniors in accurately following recipes. Magnetic measuring spoons can be easily stored and retrieved.

Steamer Baskets with Easy Handling:
Choose steamer baskets that are easy to insert and remove from pots. This allows seniors to prepare nutrient-rich, steamed vegetables without the risk of burns or spills.

Senior-Friendly Slow Cooker:
Consider a slow cooker with straightforward controls and a light indicator to signal when a meal is ready. This appliance simplifies the process of preparing hearty plant-based stews and soups.

Color-Coded Utensils:
Enhance kitchen organization with color-coded utensils for different purposes, aiding seniors in quickly identifying the right tool for the task.

Accessible Spice Organization:
Set up a spice rack with clearly labeled jars for
easy identification. This makes it simpler for
seniors to add flavor to their plant-based
dishes without the need for excessive salt.

Adaptive Seating Arrangements:
Create comfortable seating arrangements in
the kitchen, considering adjustable chairs or
stools to accommodate varying mobility levels.

Good Lighting:
Ensure ample, well-distributed lighting in the
kitchen to enhance visibility and reduce the risk
of accidents during food preparation.

2.2 Stocking the Pantry with Senior-Friendly Staples

Grains and Cereals:
Brown Rice: A versatile and easy-to-cook whole grain.
Quinoa: A protein-rich option that cooks quickly.
Oats: Ideal for breakfast or as a base for baking.

Legumes and Pulses:
Canned Beans: Convenient for quick protein additions to salads, soups, or stews.
Lentils: Quick-cooking and versatile for various dishes.
Chickpeas: A fiber and protein powerhouse for salads and curries.

Plant-Based Proteins:
Tofu: A versatile protein source that takes on various flavors.
Tempeh: Fermented soybean product with a nutty flavor.
Textured Vegetable Protein (TVP): A great meat substitute for stews and chili.

Healthy Fats:
Avocado Oil: A heart-healthy oil for cooking and salads.
Nuts and Seeds: Almonds, walnuts, chia seeds, and flaxseeds for added texture, flavor, and omega-3 fatty acids.

Canned and Jarred Goods:
Canned Tomatoes: A pantry staple for sauces and stews.
Vegetable Broth: A quick way to add flavor to soups and stews.
Jarred Olives: A flavorful addition to salads and Mediterranean dishes.

Whole-Grain Pasta and Noodles:
Whole Wheat or Lentil Pasta: Healthier alternatives to traditional pasta.
Rice Noodles: Ideal for stir-fries and Asian-inspired dishes.

Herbs and Spices:
Dried Herbs: Basil, oregano, thyme, and rosemary for flavor without excessive salt.
Spice Blends: Curry powder, chili powder, and cumin for diverse flavor profiles.

Nutritional Yeast:
Adds a cheesy flavor to plant-based dishes, providing additional nutrients.

Dried Fruits:
Raisins, Apricots, and Dates: Natural sweeteners for desserts or snacks.

Whole-Grain Baking Essentials:
Whole Wheat Flour: A healthier alternative for baking.
Baking Powder and Baking Soda: Essential for plant-based baking recipes.

Plant-Based Milk Alternatives:
Almond Milk, Oat Milk, or Soy Milk: Versatile options for cooking, baking, and beverages.

Ready-to-Eat Snacks:
Whole Grain Crackers: Pair well with dips or nut butters.
Popcorn: A light and whole-grain snack option.

By stocking the pantry with these senior-friendly staples, the plant-based cookbook for seniors can offer a variety of nutritious, flavorful, and easily prepared meals. These staples provide a foundation for creating diverse plant-based dishes while considering the accessibility and convenience for seniors.

2.3 Fresh Produce Guide for Seasonal Variety

Spring:

Leafy Greens:
Spinach and Swiss Chard: Rich in vitamins and minerals, perfect for salads or sautés.
Asparagus: A nutritious and versatile vegetable for various dishes.

Berries:
Strawberries and Blueberries: Packed with antioxidants, great for snacks or desserts.

Herbs:
Fresh Basil and Mint: Add vibrant flavors to salads and beverages.

Summer:

Colorful Vegetables:
Tomatoes, Bell Peppers, and Zucchini:
Excellent for salads, grilling, or stir-fries.
Corn: A sweet addition to summer salads.

Stone Fruits:
Peaches and Plums: Juicy and sweet for
desserts or snacks.

Fresh Herbs:
Cilantro and Dill: Enhance the flavor of
summer dishes.

Fall:

Root Vegetables:
Sweet Potatoes and Butternut Squash: Rich
in nutrients, suitable for roasting or purees.
Beets: Earthy and colorful for salads or side
dishes.

Cruciferous Vegetables:
Brussels Sprouts and Cauliflower: Perfect for roasting or adding to casseroles.

Apples and Pears:
Great for Snacking or Baking: Incorporate into desserts or salads.

Winter:

Cruciferous Greens:
Kale and Collard Greens: Sturdy and nutritious, ideal for soups and stews.
Cabbage: Versatile for slaws or sautés.

Citrus Fruits:
Oranges and Grapefruits: High in vitamin C, great for immune support.

Winter Squash:
Acorn and Kabocha: Nutrient-dense options for hearty winter dishes.
Year-Round Staples:

Bananas and Citrus:
Staple Fruits: Always available for smoothies or snacks.

Dark Leafy Greens:
Kale and Spinach: Provide consistent nutritional benefits year-round.

Cruciferous Veggies:
Broccoli and Cauliflower: Versatile and available in various seasons.

Tips for Seniors:
Pre-cut and Washed Options: Look for pre-cut or pre-washed produce to save preparation time.

Frozen Varieties: Consider frozen fruits and vegetables for convenience and extended shelf life.

By incorporating seasonal variety into the plant-based diet cookbook for seniors, the recipes can showcase fresh, locally available produce, ensuring a diverse and nutritious array of meals throughout the year. This approach not only supports health but also adds excitement and flavor to their plant-based culinary journey.

CHAPTER THREE

3 Energizing Breakfasts

An Energizing Breakfasts cookbook tailored for seniors on a plant-based diet focuses on nutrient-rich, easily digestible options. Recipes might include whole grains like quinoa or oats, fruits for vitamins, and plant-based proteins such as tofu or legumes to support muscle health. Consider incorporating nuts and seeds for added omega-3 fatty acids and energy. Smoothies with leafy greens, berries, and plant-based protein powders can also be a convenient and nutritious option. Emphasizing variety ensures seniors receive a wide range of essential nutrients crucial for overall well-being.

3.1 Morning Glory Smoothie Bowl

Ingredients:

Base:
1 cup of leafy greens (spinach or kale)
1 frozen banana
1/2 cup frozen berries (blueberries or strawberries)
1/2 cup unsweetened almond milk

Toppings:
1/4 cup granola for crunch
1 tablespoon chia seeds for omega-3s
Handful of sliced almonds for added protein
Fresh fruit slices (kiwi, berries, or mango)
Drizzle of agave or maple syrup for sweetness (optional).

Instructions:

Blend the Base:
In a blender, combine the leafy greens, frozen banana, frozen berries, and almond milk. Blend until smooth, creating a thick and vibrant smoothie base.

Transfer to a Bowl: Transfer the smoothie onto a bowl, making sure the surface is equal and smooth.

Add Toppings:
Sprinkle granola for texture, chia seeds for omega-3 fatty acids, and sliced almonds for an extra protein boost. Arrange fresh fruit slices on top for added vitamins and antioxidants.

Drizzle Sweetness (Optional):
If desired, drizzle a small amount of agave or maple syrup over the bowl for a touch of sweetness.

Benefits:

Nutrient-Rich Greens: Leafy greens like spinach or kale provide essential vitamins and minerals crucial for senior health, including calcium and vitamin K for bone health.

Antioxidant-Packed Berries: Frozen berries contribute antioxidants that support cognitive function and help combat oxidative stress associated with aging.

Omega-3 Fatty Acids: Chia seeds and almonds add a dose of omega-3s, supporting heart health and reducing inflammation.

Natural Sweetness: The natural sugars from banana and berries offer a sweet flavor without the need for added sugars, making it a diabetic-friendly option.

Texture and Satiety: Toppings like granola and almonds provide a satisfying crunch, while chia seeds add a pleasant texture and promote a feeling of fullness.

Customization Tips:
Encourage seniors to personalize their Morning Glory Smoothie Bowl by experimenting with different greens, fruits, or toppings. Suggest alternatives based on individual preferences and dietary restrictions.

Conclusion:
Highlight the Morning Glory Smoothie Bowl as a visually appealing, tasty, and nutrient-dense breakfast option that aligns perfectly with the plant-based journey for seniors. Emphasize its versatility and how it contributes to sustained energy and well-being throughout the day.

3.2 Chia Seed Pudding With Berries

Mixture: 1/3 cup chia seeds
One and a half cups plant-based milk (almond,
coconut, or any other type you want)
Two tablespoons of agave nectar or maple
syrup, or to taste
One tsp vanilla essence
A small amount of salt
Raspberries, blueberries, and strawberries
fresh for garnish.

Guidelines:

Preparing the Base: Mix plant-based milk and
chia seeds together in a bowl.
Make sure all of the chia seeds are well mixed
into the liquid by giving it a good stir.
For sweetness, add agave nectar or maple
syrup, according to your preference.

Add a bit of salt to improve the overall flavor
and vanilla essence for a hint of flavor.
Be sure to thoroughly mix all the components
together.

Setting and Refrigerating: Let the mixture sit
for at least 15 minutes, stirring every few
minutes for the first hour. Once well combined,
cover the bowl and chill for at least 4 hours or
better yet, overnight. This allows the chia
seeds to absorb the liquid and form a
pudding-like consistency. The final step is to
give the pudding a good stir to break up any
clumps and achieve a smooth texture. Finally,
taste the pudding and adjust the sweetness if
needed.

Berry Topping:
Wash and prepare an assortment of fresh
berries.
When ready to serve, spoon the chia seed
pudding into individual bowls or jars.
Top each serving generously with the fresh
berries, arranging them for a visually appealing
presentation.

Presentation:
Garnish with additional mint leaves or a
sprinkle of shredded coconut if desired.
Serve chilled and enjoy the delightful
combination of creamy chia pudding and
vibrant, antioxidant-rich berries.

This Chia Seed Pudding With Berries not only
caters to the dietary needs of seniors following
a plant-based lifestyle but also ensures a
visually appealing and tasty treat. It provides
essential nutrients and can be easily adjusted
to meet individual preferences for sweetness
and texture.

3.3 **Savory Chickpea Pancakes**

Ingredients:
1 cup chickpea flour (also known as besan or gram flour)
1 1/4 cups water
1/2 cup finely chopped vegetables (spinach, bell peppers, onions, tomatoes, etc.)
1/4 cup chopped fresh cilantro or parsley
1 teaspoon ground cumin
1/2 teaspoon baking powder
1/2 teaspoon turmeric powder
Salt and pepper to taste
2 tablespoons nutritional yeast (optional, for added flavor)
Cooking oil for frying.

Guidelines:
Making the Batter: Put water and chickpea flour in a big mixing basin. Stir until a lump-free, smooth batter is achieved.

Add the ground cumin, turmeric powder, baking powder, finely chopped veggies, cilantro or parsley, salt, pepper, and nutritional yeast, if using. To distribute the ingredients equally, give it a good stir.

Resting the Batter: Give the batter a fifteen to twenty-minute period to rest. This improves the pancakes' overall texture and aids in the chickpea flour's absorption of the liquid.

Cooking the Pancakes: Add a tiny quantity of cooking oil to a nonstick skillet or frying pan and heat it over medium heat.
To construct a pancake, pour a portion of the batter onto the skillet and spread it evenly in a thin layer.
Cook the pancake for two to three minutes on each side, or until it is cooked through and the sides are golden brown.

Variations:
Experiment with different vegetable combinations or add herbs and spices to customize the flavor to your liking.
For added protein, consider incorporating cooked chickpeas or other legumes into the batter.

Serving Suggestions:
Serve the savory chickpea pancakes warm, either as a standalone dish or with a side of plant-based yogurt, chutney, or a simple salad.

These Savory Chickpea Pancakes provide a good source of protein, fiber, and essential nutrients. They are easy to prepare, versatile, and well-suited for seniors following a plant-based diet. Adjust the seasoning and vegetable choices based on individual preferences for a satisfying and nutritious meal.

CHAPTER FOUR

4 Wholesome Lunches and Satisfying Salads

Here's a detailed explanation for creating wholesome lunches and satisfying salads tailored for a plant-based diet in a cookbook designed for seniors:

Ideas for Healthy Lunches:

Quinoa and Veggie Stir-Fry: Prepare the quinoa and toss it with a vibrant mixture of veggies, such as broccoli, bell peppers, and snap peas.
For more flavor, add soy sauce, ginger, and garlic.
Because quinoa is a complete protein source, this dish is filling and nutrient-dense.

Sweet Potato and Chickpea Buddha Bowl:
Roast sweet potato cubes and chickpeas with olive oil, cumin, and paprika.
Serve over a bed of leafy greens and quinoa, drizzled with tahini dressing.
This bowl offers a balance of complex carbs, protein, and healthy fats.

Mushroom and Lentil Stuffed Bell Peppers:
Prepare a filling with lentils, sautéed mushrooms, onions, and garlic.
Stuff bell peppers with the lentil mixture and bake until tender.
A nutrient-dense option rich in protein, fiber, and vitamins.

Satisfying Salad Ideas:

Kale and Avocado Salad with Citrus Dressing:

Massage kale leaves with olive oil to soften.
Toss with diced avocado, orange segments, and a citrus vinaigrette.
The combination offers a mix of textures and flavors while providing essential nutrients.

Quinoa salad with chickpeas and cherries, cucumber, cooked quinoa, and fresh herbs combined.
Use a simple vinaigrette of olive oil and lemon to dress.
A tasty, high-protein salad that tastes refreshing.

Roasted Vegetable and Farro Salad:

Roast a variety of vegetables such as zucchini, cherry tomatoes, and red onions.
Mix with cooked farro and toss in a balsamic vinaigrette.
This hearty salad provides a good balance of grains and veggies.

Considerations for Seniors:

Texture Modification:
Ensure salads and lunches have a variety of textures to make the meals more enjoyable for seniors.

Flavorful Dressings:
Create flavorful dressings using herbs, spices, and citrus to enhance the taste without relying on excessive salt.

Portion Control:
Keep portion sizes manageable for seniors, focusing on nutrient density to meet their dietary needs.

4.1 **Quinoa Salad with Roasted Vegetables**

Here's a detailed explanation for a Quinoa Salad with Roasted Vegetables, a nutritious and flavorful recipe designed for a plant-based diet in a cookbook tailored for seniors:

Ingredients: 1 cup of washed quinoa
Two cups of assorted veggies, such as bell peppers, zucchini, red onions, and cherry tomatoes
Two tsp olive oil
One teaspoon dried herbs (such oregano, thyme, or rosemary)
To taste, add salt and pepper.
1/4 cup finely chopped fresh parsley
Balsamic vinegar, 1/4 cup
Two tablespoons of pure olive oil
one minced garlic clove
Not required: For extra crunch, try chopped almonds or toasted pine nuts.

Instructions:

Prepare Quinoa:
Rinse quinoa under cold water.
In a saucepan, combine quinoa with 2 cups of water. Bring to a boil, then reduce heat, cover, and simmer for 15-20 minutes or until quinoa is cooked and water is absorbed.

Roast Vegetables: Set the oven's temperature to 200°C, or 400°F.
Combine salt, pepper, dried herbs, and olive oil with the mixed veggies.
Arrange the vegetables on a baking sheet and roast them for twenty to twenty-five minutes, or until they are soft and have a hint of caramel.

Assemble Salad:
In a large bowl, combine cooked quinoa and roasted vegetables.
Add fresh parsley and toss gently to mix.

To make the dressing, combine the extra-virgin olive oil, balsamic vinegar, minced garlic, salt, and pepper in a small bowl.
To taste, adjust the dressing.

Combine and Garnish:
Pour the dressing over the quinoa and vegetable mixture, ensuring even coating.
Toss everything together until well combined.
Optionally, sprinkle toasted pine nuts or chopped almonds for added texture and flavor.

Serve: Before serving, let the salad sit in the marinade for a few minutes.
You can serve the quinoa salad cold or room temperature, according to your taste.

Considerations for Seniors:

Vegetable Variety:
Choose colorful vegetables for a visually appealing and nutrient-rich dish.

Texture Modification:
Ensure vegetables are roasted to a tender consistency for easy chewing.

Dressing Adjustment:
Adjust the dressing's acidity and salt levels based on seniors' preferences for a milder flavor.

This Quinoa Salad with Roasted Vegetables offers a balanced mix of whole grains, colorful vegetables, and a flavorful dressing, providing essential nutrients for seniors following a plant-based diet. The recipe is designed to be both delicious and easily manageable, considering factors such as vegetable variety, texture modification, and dressing adjustment.

4.2 **Lentil and Vegetable Stew**

Lentil and Vegetable Stew is a wholesome and comforting dish perfect for seniors embracing a plant-based lifestyle. Packed with protein, fiber, and a variety of colorful vegetables, this stew provides essential nutrients while offering a satisfying and flavorful dining experience.

Ingredients: 1 cup rinsed and dried green or brown lentils

One large onion, chopped; two peeled and chopped carrots; two chopped celery stalks; three minced garlic cloves

One can, or fourteen ounces chopped tomatoes

Four cups of vegetable broth, one teaspoon each of paprika and ground cumin

One-half tsp dried thyme

To taste, add salt and pepper.

Two cups finely chopped leafy vegetables (kale, Swiss chard, or spinach)

Two tsp olive oil.

Guidelines:

Sauté Aromatics: Heat olive oil in a big pot over medium heat.

Add the minced garlic, diced onions, carrots, and celery. Vegetables should be sautéed until tender and fragrant.

Add Lentils and Spices:

Stir in the rinsed lentils, ground cumin, paprika, dried thyme, salt, and pepper. Cook for a few minutes to enhance the flavors.

Pour in Tomatoes and Broth: Fill the saucepan with diced tomatoes and vegetable broth, together with their juice.

After bringing the mixture to a boil, lower the heat so that it simmers. When the lentils are soft, about 20 to 25 minutes should pass, covered.

Incorporate Leafy Greens:
Add the chopped leafy greens to the stew
during the last 5 minutes of cooking.
Stir until the greens are wilted and the stew
has a vibrant color.

Adjust Seasoning:
Taste the stew and adjust seasoning if needed.
You can add more salt, pepper, or herbs to suit
your preferences.

Serve Warm:
Ladle the Lentil and Vegetable Stew into bowls
and serve warm.
Optionally, garnish with fresh herbs or a drizzle
of olive oil for an extra burst of flavor.

Considerations for Seniors:

Texture Modification:
Ensure vegetables are chopped into bite-sized
pieces for easy consumption.
Consider using softer greens like spinach for a
tender texture.

Hydration:
As lentils absorb liquid during cooking, monitor the stew's consistency to prevent it from becoming too thick. Adjust with additional broth if needed.

This Lentil and Vegetable Stew not only offers a rich source of plant-based protein and fiber but also provides a delightful combination of flavors and textures. Its ease of preparation and nutrient density make it a perfect addition to a plant-based diet tailored for seniors.

4.3 **Avocado and Chickpea Salad**

Avocado and Chickpea Salad is a delightful and nourishing dish designed with seniors in mind. This plant-based salad combines the creamy goodness of avocados with the protein-packed chickpeas, offering a satisfying and easy-to-digest option for those embracing a plant-focused lifestyle.

Ingredients: 1 can (15 oz) diced chickpeas, 1 cup diced cherry tomatoes, 1 split cucumber, 1/4 cup diced red onion, 1/4 cup chopped fresh cilantro, and 2 teaspoons chopped extra-virgin olive oil
One-third cup balsamic vinegar
One tsp Dijon mustard
To taste, add salt and pepper.
Not required: For garnish, use toasted pumpkin or sunflower seeds.

Instructions:

Prepare Chickpeas:
Drain and rinse canned chickpeas under cold water. Set aside.

Assemble Vegetables:
In a large salad bowl, combine diced avocados, halved cherry tomatoes, diced cucumber, finely chopped red onion, and fresh cilantro.

Add Chickpeas:
Gently fold in the chickpeas with the vegetables, ensuring even distribution.

Prepare Dressing:
In a small bowl, whisk together extra-virgin olive oil, balsamic vinegar, Dijon mustard, salt, and pepper to create a light and flavorful dressing.

Combine and Toss:
Pour the dressing over the salad and gently
toss all ingredients until well coated.
Take care not to mash the avocados,
preserving their creamy texture.

Optional Garnish:
For added crunch and nutrition, sprinkle
toasted sunflower seeds or pumpkin seeds on
top.

Serve and Enjoy:
Serve the Avocado and Chickpea Salad
immediately, allowing seniors to savor the
freshness of the ingredients.
Consider chilling the salad before serving for a
refreshing option on warmer days.

Considerations for Seniors:

Avocado Ripeness:
Choose avocados that are ripe but still firm for
a pleasant texture.
Adjust the avocado quantity based on personal
preferences and dietary considerations.

Texture Modification:
Ensure vegetables are diced into manageable
pieces, and consider finely chopping red onion
for ease of consumption.

This Avocado and Chickpea Salad offers a
perfect blend of creamy avocados, protein-rich
chickpeas, and crisp vegetables, providing
seniors with a tasty and nutrient-packed option.
Its simplicity, coupled with vibrant flavors,
makes it an ideal addition to a plant-based diet
for seniors.

CHAPTER FIVE

5 Hearty Plant-Based Dinners

Hearty Plant-Based Dinners for Seniors are thoughtfully crafted to provide a nourishing and flavorful experience while meeting the unique dietary needs of individuals in their golden years. These dinners not only embrace the richness of plant-based ingredients but also prioritize ease of digestion, texture variety, and robust flavors for a satisfying evening meal.

Lentil and Vegetable Stew:
A comforting stew featuring brown or green lentils, a medley of colorful vegetables, and aromatic herbs. This hearty dish is gentle on digestion while offering a wholesome combination of protein, fiber, and essential nutrients.

Quinoa and Chickpea Pilaf:
A protein-packed pilaf combining fluffy quinoa with chickpeas, sautéed vegetables, and fragrant spices. This versatile dish provides a complete amino acid profile, making it both nutritious and filling.

Sweet Potato and Black Bean Casserole:
Layers of roasted sweet potatoes, black beans, and a zesty tomato sauce create a satisfying casserole. Packed with fiber, vitamins, and antioxidants, this dinner option offers a delightful fusion of flavors.

Stuffed Bell Peppers with Brown Rice and Vegetables:
Bell peppers filled with a mixture of brown rice, assorted vegetables, and aromatic herbs. This visually appealing dish is rich in vitamins, minerals, and dietary fiber, promoting overall well-being.

Mushroom and Spinach Risotto:
Creamy risotto featuring tender mushrooms, nutrient-rich spinach, and a savory vegetable broth. This dish provides a comforting texture while offering a delightful blend of umami flavors.

Chickpea and Vegetable Curry:
A flavorful curry featuring chickpeas, vibrant vegetables, and a blend of aromatic spices. This plant-based curry is both satisfying and gentle on the digestive system, making it an ideal dinner choice for seniors.

Baked Eggplant Parmesan:
Sliced eggplant layered with marinara sauce and plant-based cheese, then baked to perfection. This hearty dinner option provides a satisfying texture with a burst of Italian flavors.

Considerations for Seniors:

Texture Modification:
Ensure vegetables are cooked to a tender consistency, making them easy to chew and digest.
Offer options to finely chop or puree certain ingredients for those with specific chewing concerns.

Balanced Nutrition:
Emphasize a variety of colorful vegetables, whole grains, and plant-based proteins to ensure seniors receive a well-rounded and nutritionally rich meal.

Flavorful Herbs and Spices:
Incorporate herbs and spices to enhance flavor without relying on excessive salt, catering to seniors' taste preferences.

5.1 Mushroom and Spinach Stuffed Portobello Mushrooms

Here's a detailed breakdown of the Mushroom and Spinach Stuffed Portobello Mushrooms recipe for a plant-based diet cookbook for seniors:

Ingredients:
4 large Portobello mushrooms: Cleaned and stems removed.
2 cups fresh spinach: Chopped.
1 cup mushrooms: Finely chopped for additional texture.
1 small onion: Diced.
2 cloves garlic: Minced.
1 cup breadcrumbs: Preferably whole grain for added fiber.
1/2 cup nutritional yeast: Adds a cheesy flavor.
1/4 cup pine nuts or walnuts: Chopped for a crunchy element.
1 tablespoon olive oil: For sautéing.
To taste, add salt and pepper to bring out the flavors.

Guidelines:
Warm up the oven: Preheat to 375°F, or 190°C.

To prepare the portobello mushrooms, wash them and cut off their stems.
Arrange the mushrooms onto a parchment paper-lined baking sheet.

To sauté vegetables, place a pan over medium heat with olive oil.
Add the garlic and sauté for one more minute after adding the onions and sautéing until transparent.
Cook the spinach and sliced mushrooms until they wilt.

Prepare Stuffing Mixture:
In a bowl, combine the sautéed vegetables with breadcrumbs, nutritional yeast, chopped nuts, salt, and pepper.
Mix until well combined.

Stuff Portobello Mushrooms:
Spoon the stuffing mixture into the hollowed Portobello mushrooms.

Press down gently to ensure the stuffing is compact.

Bake:
Place the stuffed mushrooms in the preheated oven and bake for approximately 20-25 minutes or until the mushrooms are tender.

Serve: Allow them to cool a little after baking before arranging them.
If desired, garnish with fresh herbs such as thyme or parsley.

Tips:

Adjust the seasoning to meet individual taste preferences.

Serve with a side of quinoa or a light salad for a well-rounded meal.

This Mushroom and Spinach Stuffed Portobello Mushrooms recipe provides a delightful and nutritious option for seniors following a plant-based diet, offering a good balance of flavors and textures.

5.2 **Sweet Potato and Black Bean Enchiladas**

Here's an explanation of Sweet Potato and Black Bean Enchiladas for a plant-based diet cookbook tailored for beginners:

Ingredients:
2 large sweet potatoes: Peeled and diced.
1 can black beans: Drained and rinsed.
1 red bell pepper: Diced.
1 small red onion: Diced.
2 cloves garlic: Minced.
1 teaspoon cumin: Ground for flavor.
1 teaspoon chili powder: For a mild kick.
1 cup corn kernels: Fresh or frozen.
1 can enchilada sauce: Ensure it's plant-based.
8-10 whole wheat or corn tortillas: Check for plant-based ingredients.
1 cup vegan cheese: Shredded (optional).
Fresh cilantro and green onions: Chopped for garnish.

Instructions:
Preheat the Oven: Set it to 375°F (190°C).

Cook Sweet Potatoes:
Boil or steam diced sweet potatoes until fork-tender. Mash them in a bowl.

Prepare Filling:
In a pan, sauté garlic, red onion, and red bell pepper until softened.
Add black beans, corn, cumin, and chili powder. Cook for an additional 2-3 minutes.

Combine Filling:
Mix the sautéed vegetables and black bean mixture with the mashed sweet potatoes. This forms the enchilada filling.

Assemble Enchiladas:
Warm tortillas slightly to make them pliable.
Spoon the sweet potato and black bean filling onto each tortilla and roll them up, placing them seam-side down in a baking dish.

Cover with Sauce:
Pour enchilada sauce evenly over the rolled
tortillas.

Bake:
Sprinkle vegan cheese on top if desired.

Bake in the preheated oven for about 20-25
minutes or until the enchiladas are heated
through and the edges are slightly crispy.

Garnish and Serve: Take out of the oven and
give it a little time to cool.
Before serving, garnish with finely chopped
green onions and cilantro.

Tricks: Play around with the quantity of chili
powder to get the perfect degree of spiciness.
For more variation, try out other plant-based
cheese substitutes.

5.3 **Mediterranean Stuffed Bell Peppers**

Ingredients:

4 large bell peppers: Any color, halved and seeds removed.

1 cup quinoa or couscous: Cooked according to package instructions.

1 can chickpeas: Drained and rinsed.

1 cup cherry tomatoes: Halved.

1 cucumber: Diced.

1/2 cup Kalamata olives: Pitted and sliced.

1/4 cup red onion: Finely chopped.

2 cloves garlic: Minced.

1/4 cup fresh parsley: Chopped.

1/4 cup fresh mint: Chopped.

Juice of 1 lemon: Freshly squeezed.

3 tablespoons extra-virgin olive oil: For dressing.

To taste, add salt and pepper to bring out the flavors.

Instructions:
Preheat the Oven: Set it to 375°F (190°C).

Prepare Bell Peppers:
Halve the bell peppers, remove seeds and membranes, and place them in a baking dish.

Cook Quinoa/Couscous:
Cook quinoa or couscous according to package instructions.

Prepare Filling:
In a large bowl, combine cooked quinoa or couscous with chickpeas, cherry tomatoes, cucumber, olives, red onion, garlic, parsley, and mint.

Make Dressing:
In a small bowl, whisk together lemon juice, extra-virgin olive oil, salt, and pepper to create a simple dressing.

Mix and Stuff Peppers: Drizzle the quinoa mixture with the dressing, tossing to coat everything thoroughly.
Stuff the Mediterranean filling into each half of a bell pepper.

Bake: Bake the peppers for 20 to 25 minutes, or until they are soft, in a baking dish covered with foil in a preheated oven.

To serve, take it out of the oven and allow it to cool down a little.

Tips:
Experiment with adding other Mediterranean ingredients like artichokes or roasted red peppers.
Drizzle with a bit of balsamic glaze for extra flavor.

CHAPTER SIX

6 Comforting Soups and Stews

In "Comforting Soups and Stews," we present a collection of heartwarming recipes tailored for seniors embracing a plant-based lifestyle. These soups and stews are thoughtfully crafted to provide both comfort and essential nutrients, ensuring a satisfying dining experience that aligns with the unique needs of senior individuals.

Hearty Lentil and Vegetable Soup
Packed with protein and fiber, this soup features wholesome lentils and a medley of vegetables, creating a nourishing option that is easy on digestion while offering a delightful combination of flavors.

Rustic Chickpea Stew
Brimming with chickpeas, sweet potatoes, and vibrant greens, this hearty stew is a nutritional powerhouse. Its blend of textures and spices delivers a comforting meal that supports overall well-being.

Quinoa and Spinach Chowder
Blending the goodness of quinoa and nutrient-rich spinach, this chowder provides a creamy texture without dairy. The mild flavors make it an excellent choice for seniors seeking a soothing yet fulfilling soup.

Classic Tomato and Basil Soup
A timeless favorite, this tomato soup is elevated with the addition of fresh basil. Its simplicity and familiar taste offer a sense of comfort while delivering essential vitamins and antioxidants.

Butternut Squash and Apple Stew
Sweet butternut squash and apples come together in this velvety stew, offering a naturally sweet and savory combination. Rich in vitamins, this stew is a delightful option for seniors seeking a comforting yet healthful meal.

Miso Vegetable Noodle Soup
Featuring miso paste, soba noodles, and an array of vegetables, this light yet satisfying soup provides the umami flavor of miso. The variety of textures makes it an engaging and enjoyable option for seniors.

Tips for Seniors:
Prioritize well-seasoned dishes to enhance taste without excessive salt.
Incorporate a colorful array of vegetables for diverse nutritional benefits.
Opt for easily digestible grains and legumes for a gentle impact on the digestive system.

Conclusion:

"Comforting Soups and Stews" is a collection designed with the well-being of seniors in mind. These recipes not only cater to their nutritional needs but also offer a delightful culinary journey through the world of plant-based comfort foods. Whether seeking warmth on a chilly day or a nourishing option for daily meals, these soups and stews are a testament to the joy and health benefits of a plant-based lifestyle.

6.1 **Butternut Squash Soup with Turmeric**

Delve into the wholesome goodness of "Golden Butternut Squash Soup," a radiant addition to our plant-based diet cookbook crafted specifically for seniors. Bursting with flavors, this velvety soup not only satisfies the taste buds but also offers a wealth of nutrients, making it an ideal choice for those embracing a plant-based lifestyle.

Components:
Peel and dice one medium-sized butternut squash.
Peel and cut into large pieces one carrot.
One chopped onion.
Two minced garlic cloves.
One teaspoon of powdered turmeric: golden and anti-inflammatory.
A half-teaspoon of ground ginger provides depth and warmth.

4 cups veggie broth: Offers a flavorful foundation.

Creaminess is added with 1 can of coconut milk.

For sautéing, use one tablespoon of olive oil.

To taste, add salt and pepper to bring out the flavors.

Instructions:

Sauté Aromatics:

In a large pot, heat olive oil and sauté chopped onion and garlic until fragrant.

Add Vegetables:

Add butternut squash and carrot to the pot, continuing to sauté for a few minutes until the vegetables begin to soften.

Infuse with Turmeric and Ginger:

Sprinkle turmeric and ground ginger over the vegetables, stirring to coat evenly and allowing the spices to bloom.

Add Broth: Add the veggie broth and bring the mixture to a low boil. Once the vegetables are soft, lower the heat and simmer them.

Blend to Creamy Perfection:
Once the vegetables are soft, use an immersion blender to blend the soup until smooth. Alternatively, transfer to a blender in batches.

Add Coconut Milk:
Stir in coconut milk, providing a luxurious creaminess to the soup. Season with salt and pepper to taste.

Simmer and Serve:
Allow the soup to simmer for a few more minutes to meld the flavors. Serve hot, garnished with a sprinkle of fresh herbs if desired.

Tips for Seniors:
Adjust the consistency by adding more broth for a lighter soup.

Experiment with additional spices or a dash of lemon juice to tailor the flavor to personal preferences.

Conclusion:

"Golden Butternut Squash Soup" is not just a culinary delight but also a nourishing elixir for seniors navigating a plant-based journey. With the anti-inflammatory benefits of turmeric and the comforting essence of butternut squash, this soup stands as a testament to the vibrant and healthful possibilities within the realm of plant-based cooking.

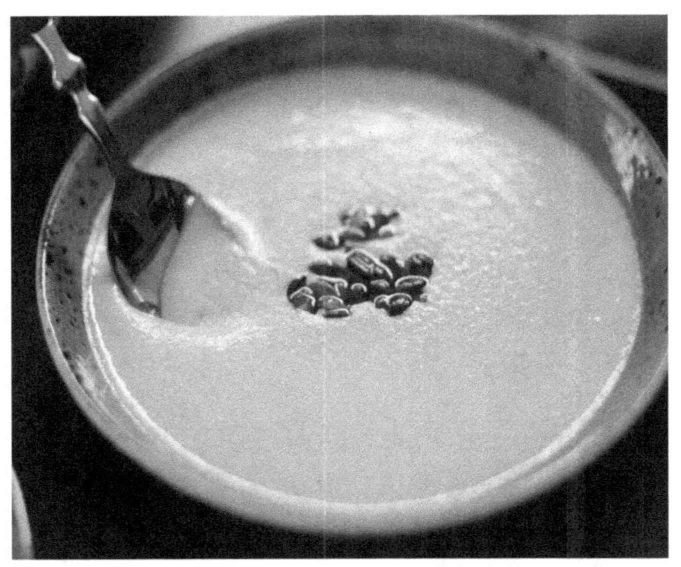

Butternut Squash Soup with Turmeric

6.2 **Hearty Vegetable and Lentil Stew**

Embark on a journey of wholesome flavors with our "Hearty Vegetable and Lentil Stew," a robust addition to our plant-based diet cookbook, specially crafted to cater to the nutritional needs of seniors. Bursting with a medley of vegetables and protein-rich lentils, this stew promises both comfort and nourishment.

Components:
Rinse and drain 1 cup green or brown lentils.
Two carrots, chopped and peeled.
Chop 2 celery stalks.
One onion, chopped.
Minced garlic cloves three.
One bell pepper, chopped, any color.
Two potatoes, diced and peeled.
One can of diced tomatoes, fire-roasted for added taste.

Four cups broth made with vegetables: a flavorful foundation.
Two teaspoons of fresh or dried thyme.
Two tsp fresh or dried rosemary.
To taste, add salt and pepper to bring out the flavors.

instructions:

Sauté Aromatics:
In a large pot, heat olive oil and sauté diced onions and minced garlic until fragrant.

Add Vegetables: Fill the pot with potatoes, carrots, celery, and bell peppers. The vegetables should start to soften after a few minutes of sautéing.

Incorporate Lentils:
Stir in rinsed lentils, ensuring they are well-mixed with the vegetables.

Season and Simmer:
Add thyme, rosemary, salt, and pepper, stirring
to coat the vegetables and lentils. Allow the
flavors to meld for a couple of minutes.

Pour in Tomatoes and Broth:
Add the diced tomatoes and vegetable broth to
the pot, bringing the stew to a gentle boil.

Simmer to Perfection:
Reduce the heat, cover the pot, and let the
stew simmer for 25-30 minutes or until the
lentils and vegetables are tender.

Adjust Seasoning:
Taste and adjust salt and pepper according to
preference. Add more broth if needed.

Serve Warm:
Ladle the hearty stew into bowls, serving it
warm and perhaps with a sprinkle of fresh
herbs for an extra burst of flavor.

Tips for Seniors:
Consider using low-sodium vegetable broth for those watching their salt intake.
Customize the stew by adding leafy greens like spinach or kale for an extra nutrient boost.

Conclusion:
"Hearty Vegetable and Lentil Stew" stands as a testament to the richness and variety achievable within a plant-based diet. Tailored for seniors, this stew offers not just a satisfying meal but a delightful fusion of textures and flavors, making it a cherished addition to their culinary repertoire.

6.3 **Creamy Tomato Basil Soup**

Ingredients:
2 cans whole tomatoes: Preferably fire-roasted for added depth.
1 onion: Diced.
3 cloves garlic: Minced.
1/4 cup fresh basil: Chopped.
1 can coconut milk: Adds creaminess.
2 tablespoons olive oil: For sautéing.
1 teaspoon dried oregano: Enhances flavor.
Salt and pepper to taste: Elevates the taste.
1 tablespoon nutritional yeast: Provides a hint of umami.
Vegetable broth: As needed for desired consistency.

Instructions:

Sauté Aromatics:
In a large pot, heat olive oil and sauté diced onions and minced garlic until golden and aromatic.

Add Tomatoes: Using a spoon, split open the cans of whole tomatoes and pour them in. Add the juice for a taste boost.

Infuse with Basil and Oregano:
Stir in fresh basil, dried oregano, and nutritional yeast, allowing the flavors to meld as you simmer the mixture.

Simmer and Blend:
Allow the soup to simmer for about 15-20 minutes, letting the ingredients harmonize. Then, use an immersion blender or transfer to a blender to achieve a smooth consistency.

Introduce Creaminess:
Pour in coconut milk, stirring gently to incorporate. Adjust the consistency with vegetable broth as needed.

Season to Perfection:
Season the soup with salt and pepper to taste, ensuring a balanced and savory profile.

Serve with Elegance:
Ladle the creamy tomato basil soup into bowls, garnishing with a sprinkle of fresh basil for a touch of elegance.

Tips for Seniors:
Opt for low-sodium vegetable broth to control salt intake.
Serve with a side of whole-grain bread or a light salad for a well-rounded meal.

CHAPTER SEVEN

7 Delicious Plant-Based Snacks

1. Roasted Chickpeas:
Ingredients:
Canned chickpeas, olive oil, salt, pepper, and optional spices like paprika or cumin.

Instructions:
Rinse and dry chickpeas, toss in olive oil and seasonings.
Roast in the oven until crispy, providing a protein-rich and crunchy snack.

2. Fruit and Nut Trail Mix:
Ingredients:
Mixed nuts (almonds, walnuts, cashews), dried fruits (apricots, raisins, cranberries), and seeds (pumpkin or sunflower).

Instructions:
Combine in a bowl for a nutrient-dense,
energy-boosting mix.

3. **Hummus with Veggie Sticks:**
Ingredients:
Chickpeas, tahini, lemon juice, garlic, olive oil,
and a variety of fresh veggies (carrot sticks,
cucumber slices).

Instructions:
Blend chickpeas, tahini, lemon juice, and garlic
to make hummus.
Serve with fresh vegetable sticks for a
satisfying and nutritious snack.

4. **Whole Grain Crackers with Guacamole:**
Ingredients:
Avocado, lime juice, tomato, red onion, cilantro,
and whole grain crackers.

Instructions:
Mash avocado, mix with diced tomato, red onion, and cilantro.
Spread on whole grain crackers for a satisfying combination of healthy fats and fiber.

5. **Nut Butter and Banana Sandwich:**
Ingredients:
Whole grain bread, almond or peanut butter, and banana slices.

Instructions:
Spread nut butter on bread, add banana slices, and make a sandwich for a delightful mix of textures and flavors.

6. **Roasted Veggie Chips:**
Ingredients:
Assorted veggies (sweet potatoes, beets, zucchini), olive oil, salt, and pepper.

Instructions:
Slice veggies thinly, toss in olive oil and
seasonings.
Roast until crisp, providing a colorful and
nutritious alternative to traditional chips.

Tips for Seniors:
Prioritize snacks that are easy to chew and
digest.
Be mindful of sodium content and opt for
low-sodium or homemade versions when
possible.
Stay hydrated by pairing snacks with water or
herbal teas.

These plant-based snacks not only cater to the
nutritional needs of seniors but also offer a
delightful variety to keep snacking enjoyable
and healthful.

7.1 Hummus and Veggie Sticks

Ingredients:

For Hummus:

Chickpeas: Cooked or canned.

Tahini: Sesame paste for creaminess.

Lemon Juice: Adds a zesty kick.

Garlic Cloves: Minced for flavor.

Olive Oil: Enhances texture and taste.

Salt and Pepper: To season.

For Veggie Sticks:

Carrot Sticks: Crunchy and sweet.

Cucumber Slices: Refreshing and hydrating.

Bell Pepper Strips: Colorful and vitamin-rich.

Celery Sticks: Crisp and low-calorie.

Instructions:

Hummus Preparation:
Blend Ingredients:
In a food processor, combine chickpeas, tahini, lemon juice, minced garlic, olive oil, salt, and pepper.
Process Until Smooth:
Blend until the mixture achieves a smooth, creamy consistency.

Taste and adjust the seasoning, adding more salt, pepper, or lemon juice if necessary.
Assembling the veggie sticks:
Prepare Vegetables:
Wash and cut carrot sticks, cucumber slices, bell pepper strips, and celery sticks.

Arrange for Serving:
Arrange the colorful veggie sticks on a plate or in a snack container.

Serve with Hummus:
Place the freshly made hummus alongside the veggie sticks for dipping.

Tips for Seniors:

Texture Matters:
Ensure the hummus is smooth to accommodate seniors with dental concerns.

Hydration Boost:
Pair this snack with a hydrating herbal tea or water to promote fluid intake.

Portion Control:
Use small, manageable portions to make snacking convenient for seniors.

Conclusion:

"Hummus and Veggie Sticks" epitomize the perfect balance between delightful taste and nutritional goodness. Tailored for seniors exploring the benefits of a plant-based diet, this snack not only satisfies cravings but also introduces a spectrum of textures and flavors that contribute to overall well-being. Enjoy this wholesome combination as a guilt-free indulgence that aligns with your health goals.

7.2 **Roasted Chickpeas with Herbs**

Roasted Chickpeas with Herbs is a nutritious and flavorful option for a plant-based diet, particularly suitable for seniors. Here's a detailed explanation:

Ingredients:
Chickpeas (Garbanzo Beans): Rich in protein and fiber, chickpeas provide essential nutrients for seniors, aiding in muscle maintenance and digestive health.

Herbs (e.g., Rosemary, Thyme, Oregano): Herbs add flavor without extra calories and offer anti-inflammatory properties, benefiting overall health.

Olive Oil: A heart-healthy fat source that enhances the taste and provides essential fatty acids for brain health.

Garlic Powder: Adds a savory element and potential immune-boosting properties.

Salt and Pepper: Use sparingly to enhance flavor without compromising heart health.

Instructions:

Preheat Oven: Set the oven to around 400°F (200°C).

Drain and Dry Chickpeas: Rinse canned chickpeas thoroughly and pat them dry with a paper towel. Dry chickpeas crisp up better during roasting.

Seasoning: In a bowl, toss chickpeas with olive oil, herbs, garlic powder, salt, and pepper. Ensure even coating for balanced flavor.

Spread on Baking Sheet: Place seasoned chickpeas on a baking sheet in a single layer. This encourages even roasting and crunchiness.

Roast in Oven: Roast in the preheated oven for about 25-30 minutes or until the chickpeas are golden brown and crispy. Shake the pan occasionally for uniform roasting.

Cool Before Serving: Allow the roasted chickpeas to cool on the baking sheet for a few minutes. This enhances their crispiness.

Nutritional Benefits:

Protein: Chickpeas offer plant-based protein crucial for maintaining muscle mass, especially in seniors.

Fiber: Aiding digestion and promoting gut health, fiber in chickpeas supports regular bowel movements.

Heart-Healthy Fats: Olive oil contributes monounsaturated fats, beneficial for heart health and inflammation reduction.

Antioxidants: Herbs contain antioxidants, potentially protecting against age-related oxidative stress.

Low in Sodium: Controlling salt helps maintain healthy blood pressure.

Considerations:

Portion Control: Seniors should be mindful of portions to align with their dietary needs and energy expenditure.

Medical Considerations: Tailor the recipe to any specific dietary restrictions or medical conditions the senior may have.

Hydration: Encourage water intake to support digestion and overall well-being.

This Roasted Chickpeas with Herbs recipe provides a tasty and nutrient-dense snack for seniors following a plant-based diet.

7.3 **Fresh Fruit Skewers with Mint Yogurt Dip**

Fresh Fruit Skewers with Mint Yogurt Dip make for a delightful and healthy snack, perfect for a refreshing option in a plant-based diet for seniors. Here's a breakdown:

Ingredients:

Fresh Fruits: Choose a variety of colorful fruits like strawberries, pineapple chunks, melon balls, grapes, and kiwi. These provide a range of vitamins and antioxidants.

Yogurt: Opt for plant-based yogurt for a dairy-free alternative. It serves as a creamy dip and contributes to gut health.

Fresh Mint Leaves: Finely chopped mint adds a burst of freshness and complements the sweetness of the fruits.

Honey or Agave Syrup: For a touch of natural sweetness in the yogurt dip.

Instructions:

Prepare Fruits: Wash, peel, and cut the fruits into bite-sized pieces suitable for skewering.

Assemble Skewers: Thread the fruit pieces onto skewers in an appealing, colorful arrangement. This step can be a fun and engaging activity for seniors.

Prepare Yogurt Dip: Mix plant-based yogurt with finely chopped mint leaves. Add honey or agave syrup to taste for sweetness.

Serve: Arrange the fruit skewers on a serving platter alongside the mint yogurt dip.

Nutritional Benefits:

Vitamins and Minerals: Fresh fruits provide a variety of vitamins and minerals crucial for overall health, including vitamin C, potassium, and antioxidants.

Fiber: Fruits are rich in dietary fiber, aiding digestion and promoting gut health.

Probiotics: Plant-based yogurt contains probiotics that support gut flora and may enhance digestive well-being.

Hydration: Fruits have high water content, contributing to hydration, which is essential for seniors.

Considerations:

Texture Preferences: Tailor the fruit selection to accommodate any dental or textural preferences seniors may have.

Allergies: Be mindful of allergies and choose fruits that are safe for consumption.

Dip Thickness: Adjust the thickness of the yogurt dip based on personal preferences, making it easy for seniors to enjoy.

Presentation:

Arrange the skewers creatively on a plate, and place a bowl of the mint yogurt dip in the center. This visually appealing and tasty snack offers a nutritious combination of vitamins, fiber, and hydration, making it an ideal choice for seniors on a plant-based diet.

CHAPTER EIGHT

8 Delectable Desserts with a Healthy Twist

**Avocado Chocolate Mousse
Ingredients:**

Avocado: Creamy and rich, avocados serve as a healthy fat substitute for traditional dairy.

Cocoa Powder: Unsweetened cocoa powder adds the chocolatey flavor without excess sugar.

Maple Syrup or Agave: Natural sweeteners provide sweetness without refined sugars.

Vanilla Extract: Enhances the overall flavor of the mousse.

Almond Milk: A plant-based milk option for creaminess.

Fresh Berries: Optional topping for added antioxidants and natural sweetness.

Instructions:

Blend Avocado: In a food processor, combine ripe avocado, cocoa powder, maple syrup or agave, vanilla extract, and a splash of almond milk. Blend until smooth.

Adjust Consistency: Add more almond milk if needed to achieve a smooth and creamy consistency.

Chill: Refrigerate the chocolate mousse for at least an hour to allow it to set.

Serve: Spoon the mousse into individual servings and top with fresh berries.

Nutritional Benefits:

Healthy Fats: Avocado provides monounsaturated fats, promoting heart health.

Antioxidants: Cocoa powder and berries contribute antioxidants, supporting overall well-being.

Low in Added Sugar: Natural sweeteners like maple syrup or agave offer sweetness without excessive refined sugars.

Vitamins and Minerals: Avocado contains essential vitamins and minerals, including potassium and folate.

Considerations:

Portion Control: While nutritious, desserts should be enjoyed in moderation to align with dietary needs.

Allergies: Be mindful of any allergies seniors may have and adjust ingredients accordingly.

Texture Preferences: Ensure the mousse is smooth and easy to swallow, catering to potential dental concerns.

Presentation:
Serve the avocado chocolate mousse in elegant glasses, garnished with a few fresh berries for a visually appealing and satisfying dessert. This indulgent yet health-conscious option is tailored to suit a plant-based diet for seniors, offering a guilt-free treat.

8.1 Banana-Oat Cookies

Ingredients:

Ripe Bananas: Mashed bananas act as a natural sweetener and binder for the cookies.

Old-Fashioned Oats: Provide a hearty texture and are a good source of fiber.

Almond Flour: Adds a nutty flavor and boosts the nutritional content with healthy fats and protein.

Cinnamon: Enhances the flavor without the need for excessive sweeteners.

Vanilla Extract: Adds a touch of sweetness and depth to the cookie's taste.

Chopped Nuts or Seeds: Optional for added crunch and nutrition.

Dried Fruits (e.g., Raisins or Cranberries):
Natural sweetness and additional texture.

Instructions:

Preheat Oven: Set the oven to 350°F (175°C)
and line a baking sheet with parchment paper.

Mash Bananas: In a bowl, mash ripe bananas
until smooth.

Combine Dry Ingredients: In a separate bowl,
mix old-fashioned oats, almond flour,
cinnamon, vanilla extract, and any optional
nuts or seeds.

Combine Wet and Dry Ingredients: Add the
mashed bananas to the dry ingredients and
mix until well combined.

Form Cookies: Drop spoonfuls of the mixture
onto the prepared baking sheet, shaping them
into cookie-sized rounds.

Bake: Bake in the preheated oven for about 12-15 minutes or until the edges turn golden brown.

Cool: Before moving the cookies to a wire rack, let them cool on the baking sheet for a few minutes.

Nutritional Benefits:

Natural Sweetness: Ripe bananas provide sweetness without the need for refined sugars.

Whole Grains: Oats offer fiber, aiding digestion and providing a sense of fullness.

Healthy Fats and Protein: Almond flour contributes healthy fats and protein, supporting overall well-being.

Antioxidants: Cinnamon adds flavor and potential health benefits through its antioxidant properties.

Considerations:

Texture Preferences: Ensure the cookies have a soft and chewy texture to accommodate potential dental concerns.

Allergies: Adapt the recipe based on any allergies seniors may have, choosing alternative ingredients as needed.

Portion Control: While a healthier option, moderation is key for a balanced diet.

Presentation:
Serve these delicious Banana-Oat Cookies on a plate or in a cookie jar, making them easily accessible for a wholesome and satisfying treat. This plant-based dessert provides a nutritious alternative, incorporating natural sweetness and wholesome ingredients tailored to the needs of seniors.

8.2 **Berry and Almond Crisp**

Ingredients:

Mixed Berries (e.g., Blueberries, Strawberries, Blackberries): Packed with antioxidants, vitamins, and natural sweetness.

Almonds (Sliced or Chopped): Provide a crunchy texture, healthy fats, and additional nutrients.

Whole Wheat Flour or Almond Flour: A nutritious alternative for the crisp topping.

Oats: Add a hearty and fiber-rich component to the topping.

Coconut Sugar or Maple Syrup: Natural sweeteners for the filling and topping.

Coconut Oil or Vegan Butter: Contributes to a crisp and golden topping.

Cinnamon: Enhances flavor without excessive use of sugar.

Instructions:

Preheat Oven: Set the oven to 350°F (175°C).

Get the berries ready: After the berries have been cleaned and hulled, combine them with a tiny bit of maple syrup or coconut sugar. The berries should be put in a baking dish.

Prepare Topping: In a bowl, combine sliced or chopped almonds, whole wheat or almond flour, oats, coconut sugar or maple syrup, melted coconut oil or vegan butter, and a pinch of cinnamon. Mix until crumbly.

Layer Topping: Evenly distribute the crisp topping over the prepared berries in the baking dish.

Bake: Place the dish in the preheated oven and bake for approximately 25-30 minutes, or until the topping is golden brown and the berries are bubbling.

Cool: Allow the berry and almond crisp to cool for a few minutes before serving.

Nutritional Benefits:

Antioxidant-Rich Berries: Berries provide a spectrum of antioxidants beneficial for overall health.

Healthy Fats: Almonds and coconut oil contribute healthy fats, supporting heart health.

Fiber: Whole wheat flour, oats, and berries add dietary fiber, promoting digestive health.

Minimized Added Sugar: Coconut sugar or maple syrup offer sweetness with a lower glycemic index compared to refined sugars.

Considerations:

Allergies: Adjust the recipe based on any nut or gluten allergies seniors may have.

Texture Preferences: Ensure the crisp topping strikes a balance between crunchy and easy to chew.

Serving Size: Practice moderation to align with dietary needs while enjoying this nutrient-rich dessert.

Presentation:
Serve the Berry and Almond Crisp warm, either on its own or with a scoop of plant-based ice cream. This dessert offers a delightful combination of flavors and textures, making it a wholesome treat for seniors on a plant-based diet.

8.3 Dark Chocolate Avocado Mousse

Dark Chocolate Avocado Mousse, tailored for seniors on a plant-based diet, is a delectable dessert that combines creamy avocados with rich dark chocolate. Here's a detailed explanation of the preparation and nutritional aspects:

Ingredients:

Ripe avocados: Avocados serve as the base, providing a smooth and creamy texture. They are a great source of heart-healthy monounsaturated fats, which can support cardiovascular health in seniors.

Dark chocolate: High-quality dark chocolate with at least 70% cocoa content is used for its rich flavor and antioxidant properties. Antioxidants, such as flavonoids in dark chocolate, may have potential benefits for overall well-being.

Sweetener: Depending on preference, a natural sweetener like maple syrup or agave nectar can be added to enhance sweetness without relying on refined sugars.

Vanilla extract: A small amount of vanilla extract can contribute to the overall flavor profile, adding a subtle sweetness.

Optional toppings: Seniors can customize their mousse with toppings like fresh berries, chopped nuts, or a sprinkle of cocoa powder for added texture and visual appeal.

Preparation:

Avocado preparation: Peel and pit the ripe avocados. Ensure they are soft and ripe for a smoother texture. Place them in a blender or food processor.

Chocolate melting: Melt the dark chocolate using a double boiler or microwave, being careful not to burn it. Add the melted chocolate to the blender with the avocados.

Blending: Blend the avocados and chocolate until a smooth and velvety consistency is achieved. Taste and adjust sweetness by adding the preferred sweetener gradually.

Flavor enhancement: Add a splash of vanilla extract for an extra layer of flavor. Blend again to incorporate the vanilla.

Chill: Transfer the mousse into serving bowls or ramekins and refrigerate for at least a couple of hours, allowing it to set and develop its rich flavor.

Serve: Once chilled, serve the Dark Chocolate Avocado Mousse with optional toppings. The result is a decadent dessert that satisfies sweet cravings while aligning with plant-based dietary preferences.

Nutritional Highlights:

Monounsaturated Fats: Avocados contribute heart-healthy monounsaturated fats, which may support cardiovascular health in seniors.

Antioxidants: Dark chocolate is rich in antioxidants, potentially offering benefits for overall well-being and cognitive function.

Vitamins and Minerals: Avocados provide essential vitamins and minerals, such as potassium and vitamin K, contributing to bone health and overall vitality.

CHAPTER NINE

9 Beverages to Hydrate and Refresh

Herbal Teas:
Chamomile, peppermint, or hibiscus teas are caffeine-free options that provide hydration along with potential health benefits. Chamomile can aid digestion, while peppermint may soothe the stomach.

Coconut Water:
A natural electrolyte-rich beverage, coconut water is not only hydrating but also a good source of potassium, making it beneficial for seniors' overall health.

Infused Water:
Create refreshing infused water by adding slices of fruits like cucumber, lemon, lime, or berries to water. This adds a burst of flavor without added sugars or artificial ingredients.

Vegetable Juices:
Freshly squeezed vegetable juices, such as celery or cucumber juice, provide hydration along with essential vitamins and minerals. These juices are light and can be customized to suit taste preferences.

Smoothies:
Blend together a plant-based smoothie with ingredients like spinach, kale, fruits, and a liquid base such as almond milk or coconut water. Smoothies are not only hydrating but also offer a nutritious boost.

Green Tea: Rich in antioxidants and low in caffeine, green tea is a refreshing beverage that may offer a number of health advantages. It can be consumed either way, hot or cold, according to taste.

Homemade Iced Herbal Infusions:
Brew herbal teas like mint or rooibos, let them cool, and serve over ice. This provides a flavorful and hydrating alternative to sugary iced teas.

Almond Milk or Oat Milk:
Non-dairy milk alternatives like almond or oat milk can be hydrating and are often fortified with vitamins like vitamin D and calcium, supporting bone health.

Sparkling Water with Citrus:
Carbonated water with a squeeze of lemon, lime, or orange provides a fizzy, refreshing drink without added sugars or artificial sweeteners.

Lemonade with Stevia:
Prepare a naturally sweetened lemonade using stevia as a sugar substitute. This offers a satisfyingly sweet and hydrating beverage without the excess calories.

It's important for seniors on a plant-based diet to stay well-hydrated, and these beverage options not only provide hydration but also offer additional nutrients and flavors without relying on animal products. Always consider individual preferences and dietary restrictions when selecting beverages for seniors.

9.1 **Green Tea and Ginger Infusion**

A Green Tea and Ginger Infusion is a flavorful and healthful beverage option for seniors on a plant-based diet. Here's a simple way to prepare it:

Ingredients:

Green Tea Bags:
Choose high-quality green tea bags, preferably organic, to ensure a pure and clean flavor. Green tea is rich in antioxidants and offers potential health benefits.

Fresh Ginger:
Peel and thinly slice or grate fresh ginger. Ginger adds a spicy and warming element to the infusion, along with its potential anti-inflammatory and digestive benefits.

Water:

Use clean, filtered water to make the infusion.

Optional Sweetener:

If desired, a natural sweetener like stevia, agave nectar, or honey can be added, though it's best to keep it minimal to maintain a health-conscious beverage.

Getting ready:

Boil Water: Use a kettle or the burner to bring water to a rolling boil.

Steep Green Tea:

Place green tea bags in a teapot or a heatproof container. Pour the hot water over the tea bags and let them steep for about 3-5 minutes. Adjust the steeping time based on personal preference for tea strength.

Add Ginger:
Add the sliced or grated fresh ginger to the steeped green tea. Allow it to infuse for an additional 5 minutes or longer, depending on how pronounced you want the ginger flavor to be.

Remove the tea bags and ginger from the infusion before straining and serving. Filter the liquid if required. Transfer the infusion of tea into mugs or cups.

Optional Sweetening:
If desired, add a small amount of natural sweetener and stir. Adjust sweetness to taste. Serve Hot or Cold:

This infusion can be enjoyed hot or cold. If serving cold, refrigerate the infusion and add ice cubes before serving.

Benefits:
Antioxidants: Green tea is rich in antioxidants that may contribute to overall health and well-being.

Digestive Aid: Ginger is known for its potential digestive benefits, which can be especially beneficial for seniors.

Hydration: Staying well-hydrated is crucial, and this infusion provides a hydrating option with added flavor.

This Green Tea and Ginger Infusion not only aligns with a plant-based diet but also offers a refreshing and health-conscious beverage option for seniors.

9.2 **Citrus Mint Detox Water**

Ingredients:

Citrus Fruits:
Select a combination of citrus fruits like lemons, limes, and oranges. Citrus fruits are rich in vitamin C and add a refreshing, tangy flavor.

Fresh Mint Leaves:
Use fresh mint leaves to enhance the flavor of the detox water. Mint not only provides a cooling sensation but may also aid digestion.

Sliced Cucumber: To add a gentle, hydrating element to the water, thinly slice the cucumber. Cucumbers have a high water content and few calories.

Filtered Water:
Ensure the water used is clean and filtered for the best taste.

Preparation:

Wash and Slice Citrus:
Wash the citrus fruits thoroughly. Slice them
into thin rounds or wedges, keeping the peel
for added flavor.

Prepare Mint Leaves:
Wash the mint leaves and bruise them slightly
to release their aroma. This can be done by
gently crushing the leaves with your hands.

Slice Cucumber:
Wash and thinly slice the cucumber.

Combine Ingredients:
In a large pitcher, combine the sliced citrus
fruits, mint leaves, and cucumber slices.

Add Water:
Pour filtered water into the pitcher, covering the
ingredients. Adjust the amount of water based
on your desired concentration of flavors.

Refrigerate:
Allow the detox water to chill in the refrigerator
for at least a couple of hours, or preferably
overnight. This allows the flavors to infuse into
the water.

Serve Chilled:
Once infused, serve the Citrus Mint Detox
Water over ice in glasses. Optionally, you can
garnish with additional mint leaves or citrus
slices for a visually appealing presentation.

Benefits:

Hydration: The combination of citrus fruits and
cucumber provides a hydrating and refreshing
beverage, crucial for seniors to maintain overall
health.

Vitamin C: Citrus fruits are abundant in vitamin C, which supports the immune system and skin health.

Digestive Support: Mint may aid digestion, making this detox water a gentle and pleasant way to promote digestive wellness.

Low-Calorie Option: Detox water is a low-calorie alternative to sugary beverages, aligning with a health-conscious, plant-based diet.

This Citrus Mint Detox Water offers seniors a flavorful and nutritious option to stay hydrated while enjoying the benefits of vitamin-rich fruits and digestive-friendly mint. It's a versatile and visually appealing addition to a plant-based diet cookbook for seniors.

9.3 **Plant-Powered Smoothie Creations**

Ingredients:

Leafy Greens:
Include nutrient-dense greens such as spinach, kale, or Swiss chard. These provide vitamins, minerals, and fiber.

Plant-Based Protein:
Opt for protein sources like silken tofu, plant-based protein powder, or hemp seeds to ensure seniors meet their protein needs.

Fruits:
Use a variety of fruits such as berries, bananas, mangoes, or pineapples. Fruits add natural sweetness and contribute essential vitamins.

Liquid Base:
Choose a plant-based liquid like almond milk, coconut water, or a dairy-free yogurt for a creamy texture.

Healthy Fats:
Incorporate sources of healthy fats like avocados, chia seeds, or flaxseeds. These contribute to satiety and provide essential omega-3 fatty acids.

Flavor Enhancers:
Experiment with flavor enhancers like ginger, cinnamon, or vanilla extract to add depth and complexity to the smoothie.

Optional Sweeteners:
If additional sweetness is desired, use natural sweeteners such as maple syrup, agave nectar, or dates. Keep these to a minimum for a health-conscious approach.

Ice or Frozen Ingredients:
Add ice cubes or frozen fruits to achieve a
chilled and refreshing consistency.

Creation Steps:

Leafy Greens First:
Start by placing leafy greens at the bottom of
the blender. This ensures they are
well-blended and don't leave a chunky texture.

Protein Boost:
Add the chosen plant-based protein source.
This is crucial for seniors to maintain muscle
health and overall well-being.

Fruit Variety:
Incorporate a mix of fruits for a balance of
flavors and nutrients. Berries add antioxidants,
while bananas contribute creaminess.

Liquid Base:
Pour in the plant-based liquid of choice. Adjust the quantity based on the desired thickness of the smoothie.

Healthy Fats:
Include sources of healthy fats for a satisfying texture and nutritional benefits. Avocado, chia seeds, or flaxseeds work well.

Flavor Enhancers: To improve the flavor profile, add ginger, cinnamon, or vanilla extract. Adapt the amounts to your own personal tastes.

Optional Sweeteners: Use natural sweeteners sparingly if necessary. After tasting the smoothie, adjust the sweetness.

Blend Until Smooth: Process all the ingredients in a blender until a creamy, smooth consistency is reached. If extra liquid is needed, add it to adjust the thickness.

Serve Immediately:
Pour the smoothie into glasses and serve immediately. Garnish with additional fruits or a sprinkle of seeds for visual appeal.

Benefits:
Nutrient Density: Plant-powered smoothies offer a concentrated source of vitamins, minerals, and antioxidants.

Hydration: The liquid base ensures seniors stay hydrated while enjoying a tasty beverage.

Digestive Health: Fiber from fruits and leafy greens supports digestive health.

Customizable: Seniors can customize smoothies based on taste preferences and dietary needs.

These Plant-Powered Smoothie Creations provide seniors with a delicious and nutritious option that aligns with their plant-based diet, offering a variety of essential nutrients in a convenient and enjoyable form.

CHAPTER TEN

10 Special Occasions and Entertaining

Celebrating special occasions with a plant-based diet for seniors can be a delightful and flavorful experience. Here's how to curate a collection of recipes for a plant-based diet cookbook tailored for such occasions:

Appetizers:
Stuffed Mushrooms: Create a savory filling using breadcrumbs, herbs, and plant-based cheese.
Vegan Bruschetta: Top toasted whole-grain bread with diced tomatoes, garlic, and fresh basil.

Main Courses:
Roasted Vegetable Tart: Layer roasted vegetables on a whole-grain pastry for an elegant centerpiece.
Quinoa-Stuffed Peppers: Stuff bell peppers with a quinoa and vegetable mix, baked to perfection.

Side Dishes:
Mashed Sweet Potatoes: Elevate this classic side dish with a hint of maple syrup and a sprinkle of cinnamon.
Garlic Roasted Brussels Sprouts: Roast Brussels sprouts with garlic and olive oil for a flavorful side.

Salads:
Kale and Pomegranate Salad: Combine nutrient-rich kale with juicy pomegranate seeds and a citrusy vinaigrette.
Mango Avocado Salad: Create a refreshing mix of ripe mango, creamy avocado, and mixed greens.

Desserts:

Chocolate Avocado Mousse Cake: A decadent yet healthy dessert that combines the richness of chocolate and the creaminess of avocados.

Berry Parfait: Layer berries with non-dairy yogurt and granola for a visually appealing and tasty treat.

Beverages:

Herb-Infused Sparkling Water: Create a refreshing drink with sparkling water, herbs like mint or basil, and citrus slices.

Non-Alcoholic Sangria: Mix together a medley of fruits in fruit juice for a festive, alcohol-free sangria.

Tips for Hosting:

Menu Variety: Ensure a diverse menu that caters to various tastes and dietary preferences.

Presentation: Pay attention to the visual appeal of dishes, using vibrant colors and creative plating.

Interactive Elements: Consider DIY stations like a make-your-own salad bar or a topping bar for desserts.

Inform Guests: Clearly communicate that the celebration will feature plant-based dishes, ensuring guests are aware and prepared.

Celebration Cakes:
Vegan Carrot Cake: Moist and flavorful, topped with dairy-free cream cheese frosting.

Coconut Raspberry Cupcakes: Light, fluffy cupcakes with a burst of raspberry flavor.

Special Touches:
Fresh Flowers: Decorate the table with fresh flowers for a touch of elegance.

Candles: Create a warm and inviting ambiance with candles or fairy lights.

Menu Planning:
Balance Flavors: Ensure a balance of sweet, savory, and tangy flavors throughout the menu.

Consider Allergies: Account for any allergies or dietary restrictions of guests when planning the menu.

Creating a plant-based cookbook for seniors on special occasions is about crafting flavorful, visually appealing dishes that celebrate the joy of shared meals and the health benefits of a plant-based lifestyle.

10.1 **Plant-Based Options for Celebrations**

Celebrating special occasions with plant-based options offers seniors a delightful and health-conscious experience. Here's a guide to crafting a celebratory menu:

Appetizers:
Stuffed Grape Leaves: Filled with seasoned rice, pine nuts, and herbs, served with a lemony dipping sauce.
Vegetable Spring Rolls: Packed with colorful veggies and served with a tasty dipping sauce.

Principal Courses:
eggplant Lasagna: Made with layers of roasted eggplant, plant-based mozzarella, and marinara sauce.
Curry with Chickpeas and Spinach: A tasty curry made with aromatic spices, spinach, and chickpeas.

Side Dishes:
Quinoa Salad with Roasted Vegetables: A protein-rich salad featuring quinoa, roasted veggies, and a zesty dressing.
Lemon Garlic Roasted Potatoes: Tender potatoes roasted with lemon, garlic, and herbs.

Salads:
Caprese Salad with Vegan Mozzarella: Tomatoes, basil, and vegan mozzarella drizzled with balsamic glaze.
Arugula and Walnut Salad: Peppery arugula, walnuts, and sliced pears with a light vinaigrette.

Desserts:

Vegan Chocolate Cake: Moist and decadent, topped with a dairy-free frosting.
Fruit Sorbet: Refreshing and naturally sweet, with flavors like mango, berry, or citrus.

Beverages:
Non-Alcoholic Mocktails: Create festive drinks with fresh fruit juices, sparkling water, and garnishes.
Homemade Iced Tea: Infuse herbal teas with fruit slices for a refreshing option.

Celebration Cakes:
Coconut-Lemon Pound Cake: A light and citrusy cake topped with coconut glaze.
Almond and Berry Tart: Nutty almond crust filled with plant-based cream and fresh berries.

Special Touches:
Festive Decorations: Enhance the celebration atmosphere with themed decorations.
Personalized Menus: Create menus that highlight the plant-based offerings, showcasing the variety and flavors.

Interactive Stations:
DIY Salad Bar: Allow guests to build their own salads with an array of fresh veggies, nuts, and dressings.
Taco or Wrap Station: Offer a selection of plant-based fillings and toppings for a customizable experience.

Consider Dietary Preferences:
Gluten-Free Options: Include gluten-free alternatives for guests with dietary restrictions.
Nut-Free Choices: Ensure there are nut-free options for those with allergies.

Educational Element:
Plant-Based Information: Include information about the benefits of plant-based eating in event materials to educate and inspire guests.

Seating Arrangements:
Mindful Seating: Consider dietary preferences when planning seating arrangements to ensure everyone has plant-based options.

Creating a plant-based celebration for seniors involves thoughtful menu planning, a mix of flavors, and special touches that contribute to a joyous and health-conscious occasion.

10.2 Hosting a Plant-Powered Gathering

Organizing a plant-powered gathering for seniors involves thoughtful planning to ensure a delightful and health-conscious event. Here's a guide to hosting a successful plant-based gathering:

Invitations and Communication:
Clearly communicate that the gathering will feature plant-based options. Include a note on invitations or event announcements about the plant-focused menu.

Menu Planning:
Diverse Options: Plan a diverse menu with a mix of appetizers, main courses, sides, salads, and desserts to cater to various tastes and preferences.
Allergen Considerations: Take into account any allergies or dietary restrictions of the attendees when planning the menu.

Appetizers:
Crudité Platter: Colorful vegetable sticks with hummus or a plant-based dip.
Stuffed Mushrooms: Filled with a flavorful mix of breadcrumbs, herbs, and plant-based cheese.

Main Courses:
Grilled Veggie Skewers: Marinated and grilled skewers with a variety of vegetables.
Quinoa and Black Bean Burgers: Served with whole-grain buns and a selection of toppings.

Side Dishes:
Roasted Sweet Potato Wedges: Seasoned with herbs and served with a vegan aioli.
Cauliflower Mash: A creamy alternative to mashed potatoes, seasoned with garlic and chives.

Salads:
Kale and Cranberry Salad: Massaged kale with dried cranberries, nuts, and a zesty vinaigrette.
Mango Avocado Quinoa Salad: A refreshing blend of quinoa, mango, avocado, and lime dressing.

Desserts:
Fresh Fruit Salad: A vibrant mix of seasonal fruits.
Vegan Chocolate Mousse: Silky and rich, made with avocados and cocoa.

Beverages:
Herb-Infused Sparkling Water: Create a refreshing drink with sparkling water and herbs like mint or basil.
Green Tea Lemonade: Combine green tea with freshly squeezed lemon juice for a flavorful beverage.

Decorations:
Nature-Inspired Decor: Enhance the atmosphere with natural elements like flowers, potted plants, or wooden accents.
Reusable Tableware: Opt for eco-friendly and reusable plates, utensils, and glasses.

Interactive Elements:
Cooking Demonstrations: Include live cooking demonstrations showcasing plant-based cooking techniques and recipes.
Tasting Stations: Set up tasting stations with different plant-based ingredients for an interactive experience.

Seating Arrangements:
Comfortable Seating: Ensure comfortable seating arrangements, considering the needs of seniors, such as cushioned chairs and well-lit areas.

Entertainment:
Live Music or Background Music: Enhance the ambiance with music that complements the gathering's theme.
Guest Speakers: Invite experts to share insights on plant-based living or wellness tips.

Takeaway Gifts:
Plant-Based Recipe Booklets: Provide guests with recipe booklets featuring the dishes served, encouraging them to embrace plant-based cooking at home.

Gratitude and Closing Remarks:
Express Appreciation: Thank guests for attending and emphasizing the positive impact of plant-based choices on health and the environment.

Hosting a plant-powered gathering for seniors involves combining delicious food, an inviting atmosphere, and thoughtful touches to create an enjoyable and health-conscious event.

10.3 **Senior-Friendly Meal Prep Tips**

Simple Recipes:
Choose straightforward recipes with minimal ingredients to make the cooking process more manageable for seniors.

Batch Cooking:
Prepare larger quantities of plant-based meals and freeze individual portions for later use. This reduces the frequency of cooking.

Pre-Cut and Washed Produce:
Purchase pre-cut and washed fruits, vegetables, and greens to save time and effort. These are often available in the produce section of grocery stores.

Frozen Fruits and Vegetables:
Keep a variety of frozen fruits and vegetables
on hand. They are convenient, have a longer
shelf life, and can be quickly incorporated into
meals.

Canned and Pre Cooked Legumes:
Opt for canned beans, lentils, or pre-cooked
legumes to skip the soaking and long cooking
times. These are versatile and can be easily
added to salads, soups, or stews.

Invest in Kitchen Gadgets:
Consider using kitchen gadgets like a food
processor, blender, or pre-chopped frozen
herbs to simplify the preparation of plant-based
ingredients.

Meal Prep Containers:
Use portion-sized meal prep containers to
organize and store ready-to-eat plant-based
meals in the refrigerator or freezer.

Meals Made in One Pot or on a Single Sheet Pan: Select recipes that call for cooking all of the ingredients in one pot or on a single sheet pan. As a result, there are fewer dishes to clean.

Prep Staples in Advance:
Cook staples like grains, beans, and sauces in larger batches during a dedicated cooking day. Store these items in the refrigerator or freezer for quick use in various meals.

Smoothies and Blended Soups:
Incorporate smoothies and blended soups into the meal plan. These are easy to prepare and offer a convenient way to consume a variety of plant-based ingredients.

Pre-Portioned Snacks:
Portion out healthy snacks like nuts, seeds, or cut fruits in advance. This makes it easier for seniors to grab nutritious snacks throughout the day.

Use Aromatics for Flavor:
Enhance dishes with herbs, spices, and aromatics like garlic and ginger for added flavor without relying on excessive salt or processed seasonings.

Diversify Protein Sources:
Include a variety of plant-based protein sources such as tofu, tempeh, legumes, and plant-based protein alternatives to ensure a balanced diet.

Adapt Recipes to Preferences:
Tailor recipes to personal preferences. If certain ingredients are challenging, explore alternatives or simplify recipes accordingly.

Social Meal Prep:
Turn meal prep into a social activity by involving family members or friends. It not only makes the process more enjoyable but also allows for sharing responsibilities.

Consider Convenience Foods:
While focusing on whole, plant-based foods is
ideal, occasionally incorporating convenience
items like pre-made plant-based burgers or
frozen meals can be practical for busy days.

Senior-friendly meal prep for a plant-based diet
involves simplifying the cooking process,
utilizing time-saving techniques, and prioritizing
convenience without compromising nutritional
value.

CHAPTER ELEVEN

11 Overcoming Challenges and Staying Consistent

Education and Awareness:
Challenge: Lack of knowledge about plant-based options.
Solution: Stay informed by reading plant-based cookbooks, websites, or attending workshops to understand the variety of plant-based foods available.

Gradual Transition:
Challenge: Difficulty in making an abrupt dietary shift.
Solution: Gradually incorporate plant-based meals into the diet to allow for adjustment and identify preferred plant-based options.

Meal Planning:
Challenge: Planning plant-based meals may seem overwhelming.
Solution: Plan meals in advance, create shopping lists, and experiment with simple, familiar recipes to build confidence and consistency.

Social Support:
Challenge: Limited support or understanding from friends and family.
Solution: Communicate dietary choices with loved ones, and seek support from local or online plant-based communities to share experiences and gain encouragement.

Nutrient Awareness:
Challenge: Concerns about meeting nutritional needs.
Solution: Educate oneself on plant-based sources of essential nutrients, consider supplements if necessary, and consult a healthcare professional for personalized advice.

Variety in Meals:
Challenge: Monotony in plant-based meals.
Solution: Explore diverse plant-based recipes, cuisines, and ingredients to keep meals interesting and satisfying.

Convenience Foods:
Challenge: Limited availability of plant-based options.
Solution: Discover convenient plant-based alternatives or prepare and freeze batch-cooked meals for easy access on busier days.

Sensory Preferences:
Challenge: Adapting to new flavors and textures.
Solution: Experiment with herbs, spices, and seasoning to enhance the taste of plant-based dishes. Gradually introduce new ingredients to adapt taste preferences.

Digestive Adjustments:
Challenge: Initial digestive changes when adopting a plant-based diet.
Solution: Increase fiber intake gradually, stay hydrated, and incorporate fermented foods to support digestive health.

Incorporate Comfort Foods:
Challenge: Missing familiar comfort foods.
Solution: Explore plant-based versions of favorite dishes or find comforting plant-based alternatives to ease the transition.

Mindful Eating:
Challenge: Eating mindlessly and not savoring plant-based meals.
Solution: Practice mindful eating by paying attention to flavors, textures, and the overall enjoyment of plant-based dishes.

Regular Check-Ins:
Challenge: Losing motivation or consistency over time.
Solution: Schedule regular check-ins with oneself to reflect on progress, set new goals, and celebrate achievements in maintaining a plant-based lifestyle.

Flexibility and Adaptability:
Challenge: Rigidity in adhering to a strict plant-based diet.
Solution: Be flexible and adaptable, allowing for occasional indulgences or modifications based on individual preferences and circumstances.

Celebration of Success:
Challenge: Overlooking accomplishments in adopting a plant-based lifestyle.
Solution: Acknowledge and celebrate successes, whether they involve trying new recipes, reaching health goals, or consistently incorporating plant-based meals.

11.1 **Navigating Social Situations**

Communication:
Challenge: Navigating social situations may involve explaining dietary choices.
Solution: Clearly communicate your plant-based preferences to hosts or fellow diners in advance, and offer to bring a dish to share, ensuring there are plant-based options available.

Menu Previews:
Challenge: Uncertainty about the available plant-based options.
Solution: When possible, inquire about the menu in advance, allowing you to plan or suggest plant-based alternatives if needed.

BYO (Bring Your Own):
Challenge: Limited plant-based options at social gatherings.

Solution: Bring your own plant-based dish to ensure there's a satisfying option available. It's a great way to share your culinary preferences with others.

Educate and Share:
Challenge: Lack of understanding from peers.
Solution: Share information about the benefits of a plant-based diet politely. Offer to share recipes or host a plant-based cooking session to showcase the delicious possibilities.

Positive Language:
Challenge: Potential negative reactions or criticism.
Solution: Frame your dietary choices positively, emphasizing the variety and flavors of plant-based meals. Respond to inquiries with enthusiasm, showcasing the enjoyment you find in your food choices.

Flexibility:
Challenge: Limited plant-based options at traditional events.
Solution: Be flexible and creative with available options, such as choosing plant-based sides, salads, or customizing dishes to align with your dietary preferences.

Express Gratitude:
Challenge: Feeling singled out or misunderstood.
Solution: Express gratitude for any efforts made to accommodate your plant-based choices. This fosters understanding and encourages positive interactions.

Celebrate Diversity:
Challenge: Social pressure to conform to mainstream eating habits.

Solution: Celebrate the diversity of food choices and explain how a plant-based diet aligns with your health and ethical values. Encourage others to appreciate a variety of culinary traditions.

Dine at Plant-Based Restaurants:
Challenge: Limited options at non-plant-based restaurants.
Solution: Choose social venues that offer diverse plant-based menus or have vegetarian/vegan options. This ensures a more inclusive dining experience for everyone.

Host Plant-Based Events:
Challenge: Limited control over the menu when attending events.
Solution: Take the initiative to host events where you can curate a plant-based menu, providing an opportunity for others to experience delicious and nutritious plant-based meals.

Embrace Potlucks:
Challenge: Uncertainty about available options at potluck gatherings.
Solution: Encourage potluck-style events where everyone brings a dish. This ensures a variety of plant-based options while sharing the joy of diverse culinary creations.

Plan Ahead:
Challenge: Unexpected food situations.
Solution: Plan ahead by having plant-based snacks or a light meal before attending social events, reducing the pressure to find suitable options on the spot.

Culinary Contributions:
Challenge: Feeling disconnected from social gatherings.

Solution: Bring a plant-based dish to share. Sharing delicious meals can be a conversation starter, and others may become curious about plant-based options.

Empathy and Understanding:
Challenge: Dealing with others' skepticism or resistance.
Solution: Approach conversations with empathy, understanding that dietary choices are personal. Share your journey positively without imposing beliefs on others.

By approaching social situations with openness, communication, and a positive attitude, seniors can navigate social gatherings while maintaining their plant-based lifestyle and even inspire others to explore plant-based options.

11.2 Coping with Dietary Challenges

Ingredient Substitutions:
Challenge: Limited availability of certain plant-based ingredients.
Solution: Explore and embrace ingredient substitutions. For example, use plant-based milk instead of dairy or tofu instead of meat for protein.

Education and Recipe Exploration:
Challenge: Unfamiliarity with plant-based cooking techniques and recipes.
Solution: Invest time in learning new cooking methods and exploring a variety of plant-based recipes. Educational resources and plant-based cookbooks can be valuable guides.

Rich in Nutrients Options:
Providing a nutrient-dense, well-rounded plant-based diet is a challenge.

Solution: To ensure you are getting enough critical nutrients, make a variety of fruits, vegetables, whole grains, and plant-based proteins a priority. To receive individualized advice, think about speaking with a nutritionist.

Meal Planning and Prepping:
Challenge: Managing meal planning and preparation.
Solution: Establish a routine for meal planning and prepping. This could include batch cooking, planning weekly menus, and dedicating specific times for preparation to make the process more manageable.

Dealing with Social Pressures:
Challenge: Social situations where plant-based options may be limited.
Solution: Communicate your dietary preferences to friends and family, and consider bringing a plant-based dish to gatherings. Educate others on the benefits of a plant-based diet to foster understanding.

Shopping Strategies:
Challenge: Navigating the grocery store for plant-based options.
Solution: Familiarize yourself with plant-based brands and products. Plan shopping lists ahead of time, focusing on fresh produce, grains, legumes, and plant-based alternatives.

Adapting Familiar Recipes:
Challenge: Adapting traditional recipes to plant-based versions.
Solution: Experiment with plant-based substitutes in familiar recipes. For example, use mushrooms or lentils in place of meat, and nut-based milk instead of dairy.

Hydration and Fiber:
Challenge: Ensuring adequate hydration and fiber intake.
Solution: Prioritize water consumption and incorporate fiber-rich foods like fruits, vegetables, and whole grains to support digestive health.

Individualizing Nutrient Needs:
Challenge: Meeting individual nutrient requirements.
Solution: Consider individual factors such as age, health conditions, and personal preferences. Adjust the plant-based diet to meet specific nutritional needs and consult with a healthcare professional if necessary.

Mindful Eating Practices:
Challenge: Overcoming cravings or habits from a previous diet.
Solution: Practice mindful eating, savoring each bite and appreciating the flavors of plant-based meals. Gradually introduce new flavors to replace previous dietary preferences.

Incorporating Plant-Based Proteins:
Challenge: Ensuring sufficient protein intake.
Solution: Explore diverse plant-based protein sources such as legumes, tofu, tempeh, and plant-based protein alternatives. Include a variety to meet protein needs.

Exploring Culinary Creativity:
Challenge: Feeling limited in culinary creativity.
Solution: Embrace the opportunity to explore new flavors, ingredients, and cooking techniques. Get creative with herbs, spices, and global cuisines to enhance variety.

Seeking Professional Guidance:
Challenge: Uncertainty about dietary needs.
Solution: Consult with a registered dietitian or nutritionist who specializes in plant-based diets. They can provide personalized advice based on individual health goals and requirements.

Mindset Shift:
Challenge: Shifting from a non-plant-based mindset.
Solution: Cultivate a positive and open mindset towards plant-based living. Focus on the health benefits, ethical considerations, and the enjoyment of exploring diverse plant-based meals.

11.3 Creating a Sustainable Plant-Based Lifestyle

Creating a sustainable plant-based lifestyle for seniors involves a comprehensive approach to nutrition, lifestyle, and environmental consciousness. Here's a detailed guide:

Diet Rich in Nutrients: Variety of Plant-Based Foods: To guarantee that seniors receive a wide range of nutrients, incorporate a selection of fruits, vegetables, whole grains, nuts, seeds, and legumes.
Protein Sources: Include plant-based protein sources such edamame, tofu, tempeh, beans, lentils, and chickpeas. Think about grains high in protein, such as amaranth and quinoa.
Healthy Fats: Consume foods high in vital fatty acids, such as avocados, nuts, seeds, and olive oil.

Nutritional Consultation:

Individualized Plans: Consult a nutritionist to create personalized meal plans, considering the specific nutritional needs of seniors, including potential deficiencies common in aging individuals.

Supplementation: Assess the need for supplements, especially for vitamin B12, calcium, and vitamin D, which can be challenging to obtain solely from plant-based sources.

Physical Activity:

Adapted Exercises: Encourage physical activity tailored to seniors, such as walking, yoga, or gentle strength training. This promotes overall health, mobility, and supports a sustainable lifestyle.

Community Engagement:

Local Farmers' Markets: Foster a sense of community and connection by frequenting local farmers' markets or participating in community-supported agriculture programs.

This encourages seniors to enjoy fresh, locally sourced produce.

Community Gardens: Engage in or support community gardens, promoting both social interaction and access to homegrown, sustainable produce.

Environmental Consciousness:

Locally Sourced, Seasonal Foods: Choose locally sourced and seasonal produce to reduce the environmental impact of transportation and support local farmers.

Reducing Waste: Minimize single-use plastics, opt for reusable containers, and practice composting to decrease the ecological footprint associated with food consumption.

Education and Empowerment:

Environmental Impact: Educate seniors about the environmental benefits of a plant-based lifestyle, fostering a sense of purpose in contributing to sustainability.

Health Awareness: Empower seniors with knowledge about the positive impact of their dietary choices on personal health, including potential improvements in energy levels, weight management, and disease prevention.

Regular Health Monitoring:
Regular Check-ups: Schedule regular health check-ups to monitor the impact of the plant-based lifestyle on seniors' well-being. Adjust dietary plans as needed based on individual health requirements.

By integrating these elements, a sustainable plant-based lifestyle for seniors can be achieved, promoting health, community engagement, and environmental stewardship.

CONCLUSION

In conclusion, " Plant-Based Diet Cookbook for Seniors" serves as a comprehensive guide to fostering a sustainable and health-conscious lifestyle for seniors. This cookbook goes beyond recipes, providing valuable insights into the nutritional needs of older individuals and offering a diverse array of plant-based meals tailored to support their well-being.

The book emphasizes the importance of a nutrient-rich diet, incorporating a wide range of fruits, vegetables, whole grains, legumes, and plant-based protein sources. It recognizes the need for individualized nutrition plans, urging readers to consult with professionals to address specific health requirements.

Notably, "Plant-Based Diet Cookbook for Seniors" goes beyond the kitchen, encouraging seniors to engage in adapted physical activities, fostering community connections through local farmers' markets and community gardens. The environmental consciousness threaded throughout the book encourages readers to choose locally sourced, seasonal foods, thereby reducing their ecological footprint.

Empowerment and education are pivotal themes, with the book enlightening seniors about the positive impacts of their dietary choices on personal health and the environment. By providing the tools to make informed decisions, this cookbook aims to empower seniors to lead vibrant, fulfilling lives through a sustainable plant-based lifestyle.

In essence, "Plant-Based Diet Cookbook for Seniors" is not just a cookbook; it's a holistic guide that celebrates the synergy between nutritious eating, physical activity, community engagement, and environmental awareness. Through its thoughtful content, this book strives to inspire seniors to embrace a plant-based lifestyle, unlocking a path to vitality, longevity, and well-rounded well-being.

Thank you for embarking on this plant-based journey with "Plant-Based Diet Cookbook." Your commitment to exploring a healthier, more sustainable lifestyle for seniors is truly commendable.

In each recipe and piece of advice, we've strived to infuse vitality into the golden years, fostering well-being through nourishing plant-based choices. Your dedication to making positive changes in the lives of seniors is a step towards a more vibrant and sustainable future.

We're grateful for your time and hope the pages of this cookbook inspire countless delicious, plant-powered meals and a renewed sense of well-being for the seniors in your life.